THIRD EDITION

Motivating People to Be Physically Active

Bess H. Marcus, PhD
Brown University

Dori Pekmezi, PhD
University of Alabama at Birmingham

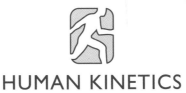

Library of Congress Cataloging-in-Publication Data

Names: Marcus, Bess, 1961- author. | Pekmezi, Dori, 1980- author.
Title: Motivating people to be physically active / Bess H. Marcus, PhD, Brown University ; Dori Pekmezi, PhD, University of Alabama.
Description: Third edition. | Champaign, IL : Human Kinetics, [2025] | Includes bibliographical references and index.
Identifiers: LCCN 2023054746 (print) | LCCN 2023054747 (ebook) | ISBN 9781718217003 (paperback) | ISBN 9781718217010 (epub) | ISBN 9781718217027 (pdf)
Subjects: LCSH: Exercise therapy. | Exercise--Psychological aspects. | Motivation (Psychology) | Health behavior. | Physical education and training. | BISAC: HEALTH & FITNESS / General | SELF-HELP / Personal Growth / General
Classification: LCC RM725 .M373 2025 (print) | LCC RM725 (ebook) | DDC 615.8/2--dc23/eng/20231129
LC record available at https://lccn.loc.gov/2023054746
LC ebook record available at https://lccn.loc.gov/2023054747

ISBN: 978-1-7182-1700-3 (print)

Copyright © 2025 by Bess H. Marcus, Dori Pekmezi
Copyright © 2009, 2003 by Bess H. Marcus, LeighAnn H. Forsyth

Human Kinetics supports copyright. Copyright fuels scientific and artistic endeavor, encourages authors to create new works, and promotes free speech. Thank you for buying an authorized edition of this work and for complying with copyright laws by not reproducing, scanning, or distributing any part of it in any form without written permission from the publisher. You are supporting authors and allowing Human Kinetics to continue to publish works that increase the knowledge, enhance the performance, and improve the lives of people all over the world. To report suspected copyright infringement of content published by Human Kinetics, contact us at permissions@hkusa.com. To request permission to legally reuse content published by Human Kinetics, please refer to the information at https://US.HumanKinetics.com/pages/permissions-translations-faqs.

The web addresses cited in this text were current as of December 2023, unless otherwise noted.

Acquisitions Editor: Andrew L. Tyler; **Managing Editor:** Chital Mehta; **Copyeditor:** Joan E.Little; **Proofreader:** Mary Frediani; **Indexer:** Nan Badgett; **Permissions Manager:** Laurel Mitchell; **Senior Graphic Designer (Design):** Joe Buck; **Graphic Designer (Layout):** Dawn Sills; **Cover Designer:** Keri Evans; **Cover Design Specialist:** Susan Rothermel Allen; **Photograph (cover):** kali9/E+/Getty Images; **Photo Asset Manager:** Laura Fitch; **Photo Production Manager:** Jason Allen; **Senior Art Manager:** Kelly Hendren; **Illustrations:** © Human Kinetics, unless otherwise noted; **Printer:** Versa Press

Printed in the United States of America   10 9 8 7 6 5 4 3 2 1

The paper in this book is certified under a sustainable forestry program.

Human Kinetics
1607 N. Market Street
Champaign, IL 61820
USA

United States and International
Website: US.HumanKinetics.com
Email: info@hkusa.com
Phone: 1-800-747-4457

Canada
Website: Canada.HumanKinetics.com
Email: info@hkcanada.com

E8875

To my late parents, Betty and Ben, for their support and love and for inspiring me to help make the world a better place; to my late colleague, Steve Blair, for being such an amazing friend and advisor; to my awesome kids, Brittany, Josh and Amber who make each day an adventure and remind me what really matters in life. To my fiancé, Chris, for all the adventures we have had and the journey to come.

—BHM

To my husband, Gary, for all the small kindnesses, long walks and beautiful children; to our beloved sons, Ian, Aleks, and Julian, thank you for bringing so much joy (and chaos!) into our lives; to my parents and brothers for their unconditional love and inappropriate humor; to Dr. Roselli for healing my heart and tennis for keeping it happy and healthy.

—DWP

CONTENTS

Preface vi • Acknowledgments viii

Part 1 Theoretical Background and Tools for Measuring Motivational Readiness 1

1 Describing Physical Activity Interventions 3
Physical Activity Recommendations 4
Definitions of Physical Activity, Exercise, and Physical Fitness 5
Physical Activity Interventions 7
Theoretical Models 8
Motivational Readiness for Behavior Change 8
Conclusion 9

2 The Stages of Motivational Readiness for Change Model 11
Motivational Readiness and the Stages of Change 12
Match Treatment Strategies to Stages of Change 15
Processes of Behavior Change 16
Conclusion 21

3 Integrating Other Psychological Theories and Models 23
Ecological Model 23
Community models 25
Individual and Interpersonal Models 26
Conclusion 35

4 Putting Theories to Work by Looking at Mediators of Change 39
Consider Mediators of Physical Activity Behavior Change 39
Factors That Enhance Physical Activity 43
Unlock the Black Box 53
Conclusion 55

5 Using the Stages Model for Successful Physical Activity Interventions 57
Jump Start to Health: A Workplace-Based Study 58
Jump Start: A Community-Based Study 59
Project Active: A Community-Based Study 61
Project STRIDE: A Community-Based Study 62
Step Into Motion: A Community-Based Study 64
Conclusion 65

Part II Applications 67

6 Assessing Physical Activity Patterns and Physical Fitness 69
Discovering Patterns of Physical Activity Behavior 70
Determining Intensity Level 71
Tracking Time 73
Assessing Fitness 83
Conclusion 87

7 Using the Stages Model in Individual Counseling 89
Physical Readiness 89
Physical Activity History 92
Psychological Readiness 92
Confidence 98
Set Short- and Long-Term Goals 100
Measure Success 102
Conclusion 115

8 Using the Stages Model in Group Counseling Programs 117
Leading a Stage-Based Group 118
Learning From a Sample Stage-Based Curriculum 126
Assessing Your Effectiveness as a Leader 129
Conclusion 135

9 Using the Stages Model in Worksite Programs 137
Building Support for Your Program 139
Assessing Motivational Readiness 140
Choosing Your Target Audience 141
Reaching Your Target Audience 142
Developing Stage-Matched Materials 142
Focusing on Moderate-Intensity Activity 144
Planning Events 144
Adding Incentives for Participation 145
Conclusion 152

10 Using the Stages Model in Community Programs 153
Assessing the Community's Readiness for Change 154
Reaching Individuals Within a Community 158
Developing Stage-Matched Messages 160
Using a Remote Approach to Reach Your Target Audience 162
Working With Community Leaders to Reach Your Target Audience 165
Conclusion 174

Appendix A: Questionnaires 175 • Appendix B: Resources 189
References 193 • Index 211 • About the Authors 216

PREFACE

Our purpose in writing this book was to translate theories and concepts from behavioral science research into a handbook useful for health professionals who are involved in planning, developing, implementing, or evaluating physical activity programs. We hope that *Motivating People to Be Physically Active* will be useful for you if you are a personal trainer, an employee at a health club or community center, a staff member at a community or federal agency, or if any aspect of your job involves helping people increase their motivation for behavior change, especially behavior change related to physical activity. We have filled this book with practical tools, case studies, ideas, and methods that you can readily use, no matter how much you know or do not know about the fields of psychology and behavior change.

You may choose to read this book in its entirety, or you may choose to read just the chapters that are most relevant for your work. However, we hope that you will become familiar with the concept of motivational readiness so that you can use this book as a reference for ideas and strategies for putting those ideas into practice. The skills, tools, and strategies presented here can be used in individual, group, workplace, or community settings.

Although the aim of *Motivating People to Be Physically Active* is to provide you with knowledge, skills, and resources for working with healthy adults, you can apply the information presented here to whatever population you work with, including populations with chronic physical or psychological conditions.

In the first part of the book, we focus on the foundations of research on physical activity interventions, tools for measuring motivational readiness for behavior change, and mediators of behavior change. In chapter 1 we differentiate physical activity programs from other programs that pertain to exercise and fitness training. In chapter 2 we introduce the stages of motivational readiness for change model, the theoretical model that serves as the foundation of much of this book. In this chapter we also discuss how to measure motivational readiness for change. In chapter 3 we discuss other influential psychological theories and models and their applications to physical activity interventions. In chapter 4 we describe mediators of change for physical activity behavior, which is what needs to change before people can change their physical activity behavior. We also describe how to measure these mediators of change. In chapter 5 we review successful physical activity intervention studies that have used the stages of motivational readiness model.

In part II we describe assessing patterns of physical activity and physical fitness, and we also look at applying the stages of motivational readiness model to various settings. In chapter 6 we describe how to measure your clients' physical activity patterns and physical fitness. In chapters 7 through 10 we discuss how to apply the stages of motivational readiness model to individual, group, worksite, and community settings. We also discuss how you can apply these concepts to specific populations. Within these chapters we provide exercises and worksheets that you can use in your physical activity programs and case studies that we hope will give you some ideas of how you might use the information presented.

This latest edition comes with a new Instructor Guide that provides a road map and activities for instructors interested in using this book in a classroom setting.

We wish you much success in your work helping people to be physically active. We applaud you for focusing your time and energy on this critically important area of health promotion and disease prevention.

ACKNOWLEDGMENTS

We want to acknowledge the many years of friendship and mutual respect that made writing this book together such a fun, pleasurable experience. Writing this book was difficult at times, especially while juggling demands from work and home, but laughter and frequent silly emails kept us "motivated". Coffee was also an integral part of the process and deserves its own round of applause.

We extend our thanks to Rachelle Edgar who always helps us with everything to keep our science and our writing on track!

PART 1

Theoretical Background and Tools for Measuring Motivational Readiness

The first part of this book focuses on the foundations of research on physical activity behavior, physical activity interventions, tools for measuring motivational readiness for behavior change, and mediators of behavior change. This part also describes the public health recommendations for participation in a physically active lifestyle and the types of activities that can be performed at a moderate intensity. We explain the health benefits of participating in physical activity as well. Finally, we describe the differences between physical fitness, exercise, and physical activity and explain the importance of theory-based interventions aimed at the promotion of a physically active lifestyle.

CHAPTER 1

Describing Physical Activity Interventions

Sedentary living is a leading cause of poor quality of life, disability, and death in the United States and many other countries. Numerous well-conducted research studies on this topic have been completed over the past 50 years, providing convincing evidence of the important physiological and psychological changes that occur during and following physical activity programs. Over the past 30 years, numerous public health organizations, including the U.S. Department of Health and Human Services (USDHHS), the Centers for Disease Control and Prevention, the American Heart Association, the American College of Sports Medicine, the National Institutes of Health (NIH), and the Surgeon General's office, have released statements regarding the health benefits of an active lifestyle and the health consequences of a sedentary lifestyle (Fletcher et al., 1992; Haskell et al., 2007; NIH, 1996; Pate et al., 1995; USDHHS, 1996, 2000, 2018). These statements are based on consistent findings from population-based studies that physical activity or physical fitness reduces the risk of cardiovascular disease in a dose-response manner. That is, those who have the greatest fitness or participate in the greatest amount of physical activity have the lowest risk. These studies also found that those who perform moderate amounts of activity or who are moderately fit also have a large reduction in their risk for cardiovascular disease relative to sedentary people. A list of the health benefits acquired through an active lifestyle follows.

Benefits of Physical Activity

Reduced risk of heart disease, high blood pressure, and diabetes

Reduced risk of cancers of the bladder, breast, colon, endometrium, esophagus, kidney, lung, and stomach

Healthy and strong bones

Better weight management

Increased energy

Better sleep

Less anxiety and depression

Lower risk of adverse blood lipid profile

Improved cognition

Reduced risk of dementia (including Alzheimer's disease)

Improved quality of life

Lower risk of falls (older adults)

From U.S. Department of Health and Human Services, *Physical Activity Guidelines for Americans*, 2nd ed. (Washington, DC: U.S. Department of Health and Human Services, 2018).

PHYSICAL ACTIVITY RECOMMENDATIONS

Data from various studies have allowed researchers to develop guidelines for the amount of exercise needed to create and maintain these health benefits. Findings from these studies led the USDHHS to develop the physical activity guidelines with which many of you are already quite familiar. First, people are encouraged to move more and sit less throughout the day. While there are many ways to accomplish this objective, examples of more specific advice from the Canadian 24-Hour Movement Guidelines include limiting sedentary time to eight hours per day with no more than three hours of recreational screen time (Ross et al., 2020).

For aerobic physical activity, which increases the heart rate and the body's use of oxygen, the consensus remains that adults should participate in at least 150 to 300 minutes per week of moderate-intensity aerobic physical activity, 75 to 150 minutes per week at vigorous intensity, or an equivalent combination for substantial health benefits. Adults who engage in 300 minutes per week of moderate-intensity physical activity gain additional health benefits. Spreading the aerobic activity across the week is ideal.

Moderate-intensity activities are those that require exerting some effort without pushing oneself as hard as required by more vigorous-intensity activities, such as running. A good example of moderate-intensity activity is brisk walking; that is, walking with a purpose, as though you were late for a meeting, trying to catch a bus, or hurrying to get out of the cold. Page 5 lists more examples of moderate-intensity physical activities.

Several studies have examined the effects of intensity level as well as the minimum length of each bout of activity. For example, several short bouts (e.g., three 10-minute bouts) of moderate-vigorous-intensity activity in a day produced similar improvements in health-related outcomes (e.g., fitness, HDL cholesterol) as one or two longer sessions. Moreover, clients may find shorter bouts easier to fit into their lifestyles. The 2008 Physical Activity Guidelines for Americans focused on 10-minute or longer bouts of moderate-to-vigorous physical activity, whereas newer guidelines recognize that bouts of any length count. Thus, both vigorous- and moderate-intensity activity have important health implications, as do both continuous and accumulated bouts of activity.

Along with aerobic activity, the recommendation is that adults perform muscle-strengthening activities on two or more days per week, involving all the major muscle groups of the body—the legs, hips, back, abdomen, chest, shoulders, and arms. Such activities can include lifting weights, using elastic bands or body weight for resistance, or anything that uses the body's muscles to work or hold against an applied force or weight.

Examples of Moderate-Intensity Physical Activities
Bicycling
Brisk walking (15-20 min/mile)
Dancing
Gardening and yard work
Hiking
Playing actively with children
Playing basketball
Raking leaves
Swimming laps

DEFINITIONS OF PHYSICAL ACTIVITY, EXERCISE, AND PHYSICAL FITNESS

Likely because they are used to the former recommendations that focused only on vigorous exercise with the goal of fitness change, many health professionals and laypeople alike use the terms *physical fitness*, *physical activity*, and *exercise* interchangeably, although their actual meanings are not the same. Perhaps you also substitute these terms for one another. You will notice that throughout this book we emphasize *physical activity* as opposed to exercise or physical fitness. We believe that the distinctions among these terms are critical; thus, we clarify what each means:

- The term *physical activity* refers to any bodily movement that results in the burning of calories (Caspersen, 1989).
- *Exercise* is a subcategory of physical activity that is scheduled, structured, and repetitive.
- *Physical fitness* is the ability to carry out daily tasks with abundant energy and vitality, which can be attained through meeting national physical activity guidelines.

The focus of this book is developing programs that help people increase their *daily physical activity* rather than, or in addition to, planned exercise. Activities such as taking the stairs more often at work, raking leaves in the yard, and shooting baskets with the kids should be included as successful outcomes of programs such as those described in this book. A person who is underactive and dislikes vigorous exercise may be more accepting of a physical activity program that encourages such strategies.

Examples of strategies for meeting the national physical activity guidelines are as follows:

- Take one 30-minute walk each day for at least five days of the week.
- Take one 30-minute walk on each weekend day and three 10-minute walks a day on at least three weekdays.
- Set a timer to remind you to stand up every hour at work.
- Walk in place while watching your favorite show.
- Walk and talk with your friends instead of sitting down to visit.
- Do three 10-minute bouts of moderate-intensity activity (playing tag with the kids, gardening, etc.) on at least five days of the week.
- Do 30 minutes of heavy housework (sweeping, mopping) on one day, 30 minutes of heavy yard work (raking) on another day, and 30 minutes of brisk walking on at least three days.

You, as a health professional, are on the front line, working with people to change their behavior. Thus, these more recent recommendations are really

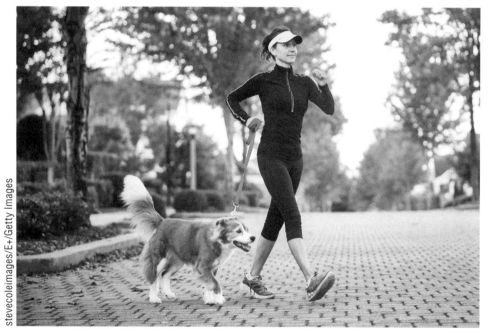

To help meet the national physical activity guidelines, engage more frequently in some outdoor hobbies that you enjoy, such as walking and playing with the dog.

written for you so that you can truly have an array of options for working with individuals, groups, or communities. We believe that most people will be much more responsive to your program offerings or individual coaching if you share with them this newer public health approach and the notion that they do not need to engage in intense, "no pain, no gain" workouts to reap the benefits of a physically active lifestyle. In fact, by giving people the choice to accumulate their activity over the course of a day or to do it all at once—for example, to do a moderate-intensity activity such as brisk walking or a more vigorous activity such as running, and to participate in physical activity at a gym, community center, or their own neighborhood—you give them the tools and flexibility to succeed at adopting and maintaining a physically active lifestyle, perhaps for the first time.

PHYSICAL ACTIVITY INTERVENTIONS

Despite the numerous benefits of physical activity and specific guidelines, only one in four U.S. adults participates in the recommended amounts of aerobic and muscle-strengthening activities (USDHHS, 2018). Moreover, the device-recorded national health and nutrition examination survey data indicated that children and adults spend approximately 7.7 hours per day (55% of their monitored waking time) being sedentary, which can lead to chronic disease and functional limitations (Matthews et al., 2003; Katzmarzyk et al., 2019). Thus, designing interventions that effectively promote adopting and maintaining active lifestyles is imperative.

Moreover, because of the many social disparities (e.g., age, income level, and education level) in the segments of the population that are sedentary, interventions that do not rely solely on costly face-to-face contact with a health or fitness professional are critical. Many people cannot afford to join a health club or community center. People in lower income brackets are also less likely to see a primary care doctor regularly than are those in higher income brackets. Thus, these people are often not well served by current facilities and organizations. This has led behavioral scientists and public health researchers to develop effective interventions that can be delivered remotely via the Internet, telephone, mobile applications, text messaging, videoconferencing, and wearable devices (Marcus et al., 2022; Marcus, Benitez, et al., 2022; Marcus, Ainsworth, et al., 2018; Arredondo et al., 2023).

Exercise training studies are typically conducted at gyms and supervised by health professionals. Psychological theory is often not the framework on which these studies are based. In contrast, the goal for physical activity interventions is to help people change their behavior and replace sedentary pursuits with active ones. For example, helping people choose to meet friends for walks or bike rides rather than lunch or coffee might be one goal of a physical activity intervention. The goal of physical activity interventions is to help people reorient their lives to include physical activity.

Physical activity professionals increasingly recognize that to keep people active, they need to help them develop physical activity habits that fit their lifestyles. For example, for a person who works at the office from 9 a.m. until 5 p.m., having home exercise equipment may be the only way to structure the environment so that regular physical activity is an option. Of course, simply having exercise equipment in the environment does not provide the motivation for the person to actually use it. For that, the person may need to learn to pair leisure activities they like and perceive as important, such as watching the news or listening to music, with the use of home exercise equipment. In this way, lifting free weights at 7:00 p.m. can be something to look forward to rather than one more thing to get through on a busy day.

Those who design physical activity interventions have also learned the importance of helping clients discover activities that they enjoy. Teaching people that activities they consider fun, such as dancing and gardening, can count toward the daily goal of accumulating 30 minutes of moderate-intensity activity is a great way to get people who otherwise might not take up regular exercise to at least consider doing so. Giving people the choice of gym-based or home-based exercise programs also has advantages. For example, studies have shown that people often do better (King et al., 1991; Jansons et al., 2017) long-term in home-based vs. gym-based programs which may be due to numerous factors (convenience, opportunities for continuous or intermittent bouts of practical activities; e.g., yard work, housework, gardening). Interventionists and program planners are becoming increasingly aware of the need to design programs that are customized to their clients' preferences and flexible enough to accommodate changes in life circumstances and routines.

THEORETICAL MODELS

Numerous theoretical models have been used to explain physical activity as a behavior, to better understand the factors that influence it, and to develop targeted strategies for physical activity intervention. For example, the stages of change approach examines people's motivation for changing their physical activity habits, the barriers that get in their way, the benefits they hope to glean from an active lifestyle, and the specific strategies and techniques for becoming more active. Applying such psychological theories to the promotion of physically active lifestyles can serve as a useful framework when helping clients meet their goals.

MOTIVATIONAL READINESS FOR BEHAVIOR CHANGE

The stages of motivational readiness for change model (Prochaska & DiClemente, 1983) provides a structured approach to examining people's motivation for changing their physical activity habits, the barriers to change, the benefits of change, and specific strategies and techniques for promoting change.

This model has great utility for those who work with individuals, groups, and communities because it highlights the need to assess both physical and psychological issues when designing programs. It also helps in the selection of strategies for behavior change that may be most useful for people with different levels of motivation to change. This theoretical framework is central to much of this book because it can help you understand how to motivate adults to be physically active.

CONCLUSION

In this chapter we have described the public health recommendations for participation in a physically active lifestyle. We have also reviewed examples of moderate-intensity physical activities and the health benefits of participating in such activities. We have explained the differences between physical fitness, exercise, and physical activity and discussed the importance of theory-based interventions aimed at the promotion of a physically active lifestyle.

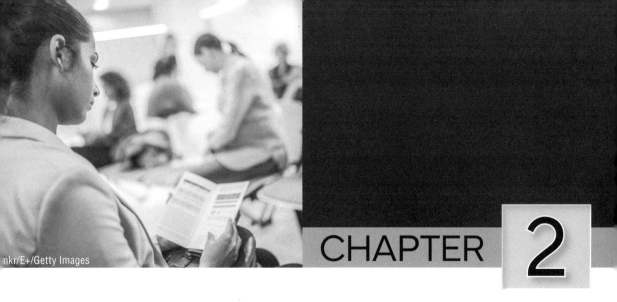
nkr/E+/Getty Images

CHAPTER 2

The Stages of Motivational Readiness for Change Model

As you may know, most Americans are not meeting physical activity guidelines (USDHHS, 2018). In the programs you manage, you may encounter people who participate in some activity, such as a Thursday night bowling or softball league or pickleball with a friend on Saturdays, but spend most of their days engaged in sedentary activities (e.g., watching TV, working at a desk). Because so many people are either inactive or infrequently active, effective programs to help them start and stick with an active lifestyle are critical.

Many of the techniques used to promote physical activity originate from psychological theories of motivation and behavior change. Behavior change can be influenced at many levels, including policy (laws), community, institutional (school, workplace), and interpersonal (family, friends), yet most work in this area has focused on the individual. Such intervention strategies address personal knowledge, beliefs, and attitudes related to behavior change. A prime example of an individual-level theory is the stages of change model.

The stages of motivational readiness for change model evolved from the work of Dr. James Prochaska and Dr. Carlo DiClemente. Initially, they studied how people quit smoking without professional help (Prochaska & DiClemente, 1983). They were interested in learning how people who are not receiving help make changes, thinking that this knowledge would provide valuable information to professionals who help others change their health habits (figure 2.1). Through their in-depth study of people who changed their smoking habits on their own, Drs. Prochaska and DiClemente learned that people moved through specific stages as they struggled to reduce the number of cigarettes they smoked or to quit smoking altogether. The model was initially labeled the transtheoretical model (Prochaska, 1979) because it was developed from many psychological theories, such as social cognitive theory (Bandura, 1977) and learning theory (Skinner, 1953).

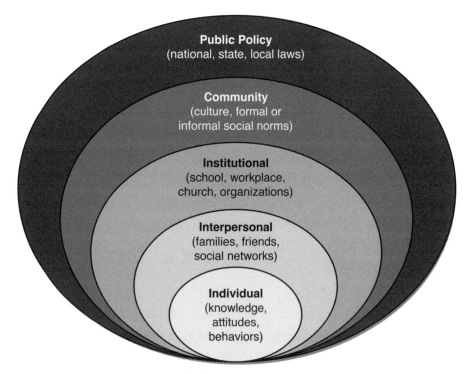

Figure 2.1 Multiple levels of influence on health behaviors.

MOTIVATIONAL READINESS AND THE STAGES OF CHANGE

Stages of change is the key concept in the model that Prochaska and DiClemente developed; thus, many people refer to it as the stages of change model. We call it the stages of motivational readiness for change model to emphasize that it focuses on both motivation for change and actual behavior change. It acknowledges that when attempting to make long-lasting behavior changes, people vary in their levels of motivation to change, from no intention to change to actually making behavior changes.

This model posits that there are five stages of readiness for change. For physical activity, the stages are defined as follows:

- Those in the *inactive and not thinking about becoming more active* stage (stage 1) include people who are not physically active and do not intend to become physically active in the next six months. This stage is hereafter referred to as *not thinking about change*.

- The *inactive and thinking about becoming more active* stage (stage 2) applies to people who do not currently participate in physical activity but intend to start in the next six months. This stage is hereafter referred to as *thinking about change*.

- Those in the *doing some physical activity* stage (stage 3) participate in some physical activity but have not reached the national physical activity guidelines (e.g., at least 150 minutes per week of moderate-intensity exercise). They may or may not intend to become more physically active.
- People in the *meeting physical activity guidelines* stage (stage 4) participate in the recommended amounts of physical activity but have done so for less than six months and may or may not maintain this level of physical activity. (They may or may not intend to, or they may or may not be able to.)
- Those in the *making physical activity a habit* stage (stage 5) have participated in the recommended amounts of physical activity for six months or longer (Marcus & Simkin, 1993).

Movement through the stages is thought to be cyclical rather than linear because many people do not succeed in their efforts at starting and sticking with lifestyle changes (figure 2.2); in other words, people move back and forth among these stages (Prochaska, et al., 1992). For example, if people are in the thinking about change stage (stage 2) and move straight into the meeting physical activity guidelines stage (stage 4), accumulating at least 30 minutes of at least moderate-intensity activity at least five days a week, this may not

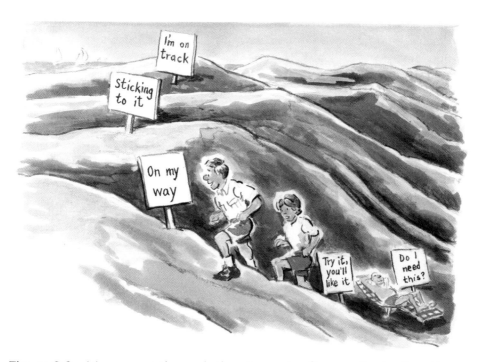

Figure 2.2 Movement through the stages is often cyclical rather than linear; people will often go back and forth through the stages.

Reprinted by permission from S.N. Blair et al., *Active Living Every Day* (Champaign, IL: Human Kinetics, 2001), 8.

result in long-lasting change. That is, if they skip the stage of doing some physical activity (stage 3), they may not be adequately prepared for the rigors of daily activity, neither for the physical demand of that amount of activity nor for the time demand on their schedule. If they develop some foot or knee pain or decide that the two and a half hours per week they are devoting to walking take too much time away from work, they may say, "Physical activity just doesn't fit into my life, so I am not going to do it." The risk is that not only will they slide back to an earlier stage, but in fact they may slide right back to the not thinking about change stage rather than the thinking about change stage.

This model is also cyclical because changing a habit often takes many cycles before attaining success. That is, people may need to make numerous attempts at behavior change before they can reach the making physical activity a habit stage (stage 5). You are probably quite familiar with the concept of one step forward and two steps back—this is often true for behavior change and may be quite frustrating for your clients.

Although the title of the fifth stage, making physical activity a habit, suggests that once people reach this level, they will maintain their physical activity for the long term, there is a strong likelihood that they will slide back to earlier stages for periods of time. This sliding back could be due to competing demands on their time, health, or a myriad of other reasons. Fortunately, research has shown that once people reach this stage, they are more likely to slide back to doing some physical activity (stage 3), or at worst, to thinking about change (stage 2), and not all the way back to not thinking about change (stage 1; Marcus, Selby, et al., 1992).

Whether a person needs to remain in the making physical activity a habit stage (stage 5) for some critical period to reduce the risk of backsliding is unknown. A few studies have proposed a *termination* stage, involving complete confidence in one's ability to exercise regularly and no temptation to relapse (Cardinal, 1999; Cardinal and Levy, 2000; Fallon and Hausenblas, 2001; 2004; Fallon et al., 2005; Horiuchi et al., 2013). While some differences have been found in self-efficacy (Fallon et al., 2005; Horiuchi et al., 2013) and relapse rates (Horiuchi et al., 2013) between individuals in termination and maintenance stages (but not pros and cons for exercise; Fallon et al., 2005; Horiuchi et al. 2013), support for the validity of a sixth stage of change for exercise remains underwhelming. It seems unlikely that participating in physical activity regularly simply becomes a permanent way of life. Even if people truly enjoy the activity in which they participate and have participated in it regularly for many years, they still need to remain vigilant to ensure that they continue. It never ceases to be an issue in their lives. This is important for program planners and those working with clients to keep in mind as they help people make short- and long-term goals for physical activity. Table 2.1 summarizes the stages of change.

Table 2.1 Stages of Motivational Readiness for Change

Stage number	Description
Stage 1	Inactive and not thinking about becoming more active
Stage 2	Inactive and thinking about becoming more active
Stage 3	Doing some physical activity
Stage 4	Meeting physical activity guidelines*
Stage 5	Making physical activity a habit

*Accumulating at least 30 minutes of moderate-intensity physical activity at least five days per week.

MATCH TREATMENT STRATEGIES TO STAGES OF CHANGE

Most intervention programs are designed for people in the doing some physical activity stage (stage 3) or the meeting physical activity guidelines stage (stage 4)—that is, people who are already engaged in physical activity. However, most of the population is not in either of these stages. Therefore, those of us interested in helping people lead more active lives need to think about other types of programs to offer those in stage 1 and stage 2. They are the ones who most need to change, yet few opportunities for change are offered to them, and they may not be ready or motivated to seek opportunities on their own.

We studied a sample of participants in a workplace health promotion project (Marcus, Rossi, et al., 1992) and classified 24 percent as in stage 1, 33 percent as in stage 2, 10 percent as in stage 3, 11 percent as in stage 4, and 22 percent as in stage 5. Other studies conducted in the United States, Australia, Europe, and Asia (even among individuals with type 2 diabetes) have shown similar percentages, with most participants in the pre-action stages for physical activity change (Horiuchi et al., 2017).

Our studies and those of our colleagues in the United States, Australia, and Europe have demonstrated that when there is a mismatch between participants' stages of motivational readiness for change and the intervention strategy used, they are more likely to drop out of the program; even if they stay in, they are less likely to reach their goals. For example, if people still in stage 2 are given information appropriate for those in stage 4, such as specific tips on exercise programs, they may disregard the materials, intending to refer to them later, when or if they feel ready to start. This increases the chances that they will forget about the information they received or decide that the program is not right for them because the material was not relevant to their level of motivation at that time. Matching treatment strategies to people's stages of motivational readiness for change improves the likelihood

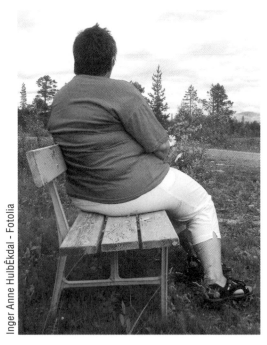

Traditional intervention programs often target those already motivated to become more physically active. Individuals in the earlier stages of change may need other types of programs.

that they will attend a program regularly, increases their chances of meeting their short- and long-term goals, and decreases the likelihood that they will stop participating in the program or stop reading the materials provided.

PROCESSES OF BEHAVIOR CHANGE

The stages of motivational readiness for change model also addresses the processes of behavior change (Prochaska et al., 1988). These processes of change are the strategies and techniques that people use to modify their behavior. The original work investigating the processes of change, like investigating the stages of change, was conducted on smokers and has since been extended to physical activity.

The stages of change explain process, and the processes of change describe *how* people change. Determining which specific processes of change to focus on with a given client depends on that client's stage of motivational readiness for change. Using a questionnaire we developed about processes of change for physical activity, we discovered that for physical activity, all the processes are important at all stages of change (Marcus, Rossi, et al., 1992). Nonetheless, it is not feasible to emphasize all processes at each contact with a person, and thus key processes are usually selected based on the person's stage (Marcus et al., 1998).

Processes of behavior change are divided into two categories: cognitive (involving thinking, attitudes, and awareness) and behavioral (involving actions).

The cognitive processes of change regarding physical activity are as follows:
- Increasing knowledge
- Being aware of risks
- Caring about consequences to others
- Comprehending benefits
- Increasing healthy opportunities

The behavioral processes of change regarding physical activity are as follows:
- Substituting alternatives
- Enlisting social support
- Rewarding yourself
- Committing yourself
- Reminding yourself

Questionnaire 4.1 for assessing these 10 processes of change (how much the client is using the process or strategy) is in appendix A. When people are in stage 2, they typically use mostly *cognitive* processes and some *behavioral* processes. People in stage 4 typically use mostly *behavioral* processes and some *cognitive* processes. These strategies and techniques for helping people change their behavior were derived from a variety of psychological theories and models and are often used in counseling (Prochaska, 1979). Table 2.2 lists ways you can help clients engage in the processes of change.

Table 2.2 Processes of Change

COGNITIVE STRATEGIES	
Increasing knowledge	Encourage your clients to read and think about physical activity.
Being aware of risks	Provide your clients with information on the health risks associated with being inactive.
Caring about consequences to others	Encourage your clients to recognize how their inactivity affects their family, friends, and coworkers.
Comprehending benefits	Help your clients understand the personal benefits of being physically active.
Increasing healthy opportunities	Help your clients increase their awareness of opportunities to be physically active.

(continued)

Table 2.2 Processes of Change *(continued)*

	BEHAVIORAL STRATEGIES
Substituting alternatives	Encourage your clients to take a walk instead of watching TV to cope with stress, fatigue, etc.
Enlisting social support	Encourage your clients to find a family member, friend, or coworker who is willing and able to provide support for being active.
Rewarding yourself	Encourage your clients to praise and reward themselves for being physically active.
Committing yourself	Encourage your clients to make promises, plans, and commitments to be active.
Reminding yourself	Teach your clients how to set up reminders to be active, such as keeping comfortable shoes in the car.

Programs based on the stages of motivational readiness for change model match treatment to the person's stage of readiness for change. For example, a stage-matched physical activity promotion intervention for people in the early stages of change (stage 1 or stage 2) might focus on increasing the use of the cognitive processes. Thus, the program might increase awareness of the benefits of physical activity and encourage people to think about becoming active. Materials designed for people in the later stages (stages 3, 4, and 5) can focus more on the behavioral processes. Such materials might encourage people to begin exercising and suggest strategies for maintaining an active lifestyle, such as rewarding oneself for reaching an activity goal or putting reminders to be active around the home and the workplace.

Working with clients to increase their self-confidence regarding their ability to become and stay physically active is helpful (Bandura, 1977, 1986, 1997). It is also usually important to help clients understand more about the benefits of becoming physically active. Finally, because behavior change is not an easy process, practitioners can also work with clients on understanding and overcoming their personal barriers to behavior change (Janis & Mann, 1977). Often, components that address self-confidence, benefits, and barriers are used in combination with the stages and processes of change in individual, group, workplace, and community programs. Chapters 3 and 4 provide more information about self-confidence and the benefits of and barriers to physical activity. The next section presents information on measuring a client's stage of change; chapter 4 provides information on measuring processes of change, self-confidence, barriers (cons), and benefits (pros).

Determining a Client's Stage of Change

In this section we describe how to measure the stages of motivational readiness for change. The flowchart in figure 2.3 is a helpful visual aid for explaining the concept of stages of motivational readiness to your clients. Studies that have looked at the stages of change questionnaire (questionnaire 2.1 in

Chapter 2 The Stages of Motivational Readiness for Change Model **19**

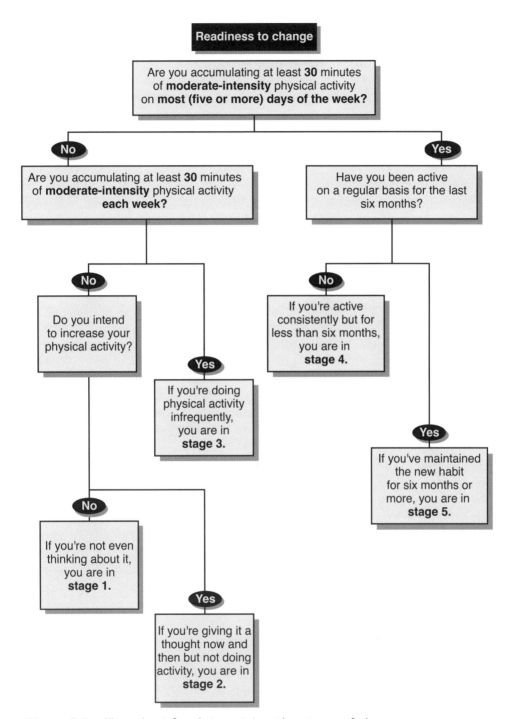

Figure 2.3 Flowchart for determining the stage of change.
Reprinted by permission from S.N. Blair et al., *Active Living Every Day* (Champaign, IL: Human Kinetics, 2001), 8.

appendix A) have found that people tend to get similar scores over a two-week period (Marcus, Selby, et al., 1992). This gives us increased confidence that this questionnaire is measuring people's intentions and actual behavior in general, not just at the time they are filling out the questionnaire. We also have found that the questionnaire is related to measures of actual physical activity (Marcus & Simkin, 1993). This is important because it means that there is a direct relationship between the stage of motivational readiness for change and the number of minutes people are physically active each week. There is also a relationship between moving forward one or more stages and increases in physical fitness (Dunn et al., 1997). You can simply copy the questionnaire in appendix A for use with your clients. A Spanish language version (questionnaire 2.2 is also available in appendix A).

Scoring the Stages of Change Questionnaire

Clients in stages 1 and 2 should have responded to questions 3 and 4 with zeros to ensure consistency in responses. In other words, clients who are inactive and either thinking about or not thinking about becoming active should answer no to questions 3 and 4, because it is impossible to not be physically active and to be physically active at the same time. Occasionally, clients answer yes to both, which indicates that they have not read the questions carefully or that they do not understand them. In this case, you should clarify the meaning of these questions for your client.

The scoring algorithm determines clients' particular stages only at the time they complete the questionnaire. However, this questionnaire has been shown to be stable over a two-week period. When clients are found to be in stage 3 (doing some activity), 4 (doing enough activity), or 5 (making activity a habit), the second question (about whether they intend to increase their activity in the next 6 months) does not play a role in determining which stage they are in at the time they complete the questionnaire. This question is used to distinguish between clients in stage 1 (not thinking about becoming active) and stage 2 (thinking about becoming active). However, your client's intention to increase physical activity in the next six months can be highly relevant for intervention planning, and thus you may want to make a note of it. For example, if your clients are in stage 3 (doing some activity) but answer that they are not planning to increase their activity over the next six months, you will probably want to ask them why they have sought your help. Perhaps they misunderstood the question. Or perhaps they came to see you only because a friend strongly encouraged them to do so, and they really have no intention of changing their behavior.

CONCLUSION

In this chapter we have described the concepts of motivational readiness and stages of change. We have discussed that this is a cyclical model and that programs have more appeal or relevance when matched to a person's level of readiness to engage in behavior change. Additionally, the processes of change, or strategies and techniques for behavior change, have been described, and the concepts of self-efficacy and decision-making for behavior change have been introduced.

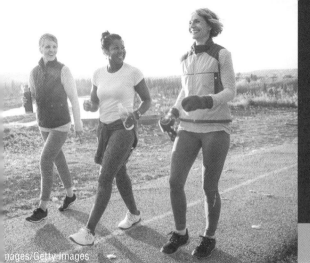

CHAPTER 3

Integrating Other Psychological Theories and Models

Physical activity includes many types of behavior, such as walking, playing volleyball with the kids, and raking the leaves in the yard. It also includes more traditional types of exercise, such as jogging and aerobics. As previously mentioned, many factors determine whether people are physically active, including self-confidence, the belief that they will gain something worthwhile from activity, support from family and friends, and whether they enjoy active pursuits and have access to safe, nearby walking paths. Some health promoters have turned to psychological theories and models to better understand the many factors involved in starting to live an active lifestyle and maintaining physical activity behaviors. Theories from behavioral science also have been useful in designing, implementing, and evaluating health promotion efforts.

This chapter describes some theories and models that can be useful when developing strategies for helping clients become more physically active. We mention several of the most promising theories because no one model seems to fully explain physical activity and the ways we can most effectively help people change this behavior. Some theories appear to be more appropriate for looking at physical activity at the personal level, whereas others are more applicable at the community level. The following section will start at the broadest level of influence (ecological models) and then narrow in focus to theories pertaining to individuals and their social environment.

ECOLOGICAL MODEL

The ecological model seeks to explain behavior and behavior change in relation to sociocultural and environmental variables. According to this approach, some environments restrict physical activities by promoting (and even demanding, in some cases) sedentary behaviors and limiting possible active pursuits (Badland & Schofield, 2005; Sallis et al., 1998). For example, many workplaces do not contain exercise facilities or walking space nearby. Moreover, the elevator is in a central location, whereas staircases are in the far corners of the building. Similarly, in neighborhood design, sprawling urban areas have been associated with more sedentary transport (car use) and time spent sitting in a car. Although we still have much to learn regarding how people's physical environments affect their physical activity, environments can be designed to foster activity by improving access to and quality of parks, green spaces, bike paths, street connectivity, and staircases that are safe, attractive, and easily accessible (Badland & Schofield, 2005; Humpel et al., 2002). The ecological model states that it is important to develop physical environments and policies that support activity, in addition to helping individuals develop personal skills, because there are multiple levels of influence on physical activity (McLeroy et al., 1988). Table 3.1 illustrates the levels of influence.

Table 3.1 Components of the Ecological Model

Components	Examples
Individual factors	Psychological Biological Developmental
Interpersonal factors	Friends Family Coworkers
Institutional factors	Companies Schools Health care facilities
Community factors	Organization of physical activity resources Activity-related events Safe walking, biking trails
Public policy	Tax breaks for healthy behaviors Laws protecting green space Better insurance rates for physically active individuals

To change physical activity behavior, the program must be implemented on multiple levels. Programs that influence multiple levels and multiple settings have the potential to produce larger, longer-lasting physical activity changes than those that do not (Sallis et al., 1998, 2018). Furthermore, it is important to customize the program to the client's physical environment. For example, an outdoor walking program in an unsafe area with few sidewalks is not likely to be successful for many residents. Past studies have found associations between physical activity and several neighborhood environment factors (e.g., street connectivity, destinations, population density, parks, safety and aesthetics; Salvo et al., 2018; Humpel et al., 2002). See table 3.2 for more examples of environmental influences on physical activity.

Table 3.2 Environmental Influences on Physical Activity

Environmental influence	Examples
Accessibility of facilities	Bicycle paths Health clubs/gyms nearby Walking paths Swimming pools
Opportunities for activities	Presence of sidewalks Home equipment Shops within walking distance Local fun runs
Weather	Temperature Daylight changes Precipitation Wind
Safety	Crime rate Unattended dogs Street lighting Traffic levels
Aesthetics	Friendly neighborhood Enjoyable scenery Green space Hills, trees

Adapted by permission from N. Humpel, N. Owen, and E. Leslie, "Environmental Factors Associated with Adults' Participation in Physical Activity," *American Journal of Preventive Medicine* 22, no. 3 (2002): 188-191, with permission from Elsevier.

COMMUNITY MODELS

When working to influence physical activity at the community level, community-based participatory research (CBPR) principles can serve as a useful guide. CBPR encourages practitioners and researchers to engage communities of interest in a respectful and collaborative manner as partners in physical activity promotion efforts (Israel et al., 1998).

Community-Based Participatory Research Principles

- Acknowledge the community's connections and common interests.
- Foster the existing community's assets, resources, and associations.
- Encourage all partners to work together and contribute to all stages of the project.
- Balance advancing public health knowledge with addressing community concerns to create a win-win situation for all partners.
- Support partners in learning from and empowering each other.
- Recognize the ongoing cyclical process, which spans from partner development to sustaining community initiatives.

- Emphasize a holistic, multi-level view of health.
- Provide key findings and lessons learned to all partners.

Another theory, diffusion of innovations (DOI), originated in the rural sociology field with Everett Rogers yet is highly relevant to the uptake and spread of physical activity resources and programs in communities (Rogers, 2003). DOI posits that targeting influential early adopters (e.g., involving community leaders) and highlighting attributes of physical activity that the target group finds compelling (e.g., chronic disease prevention, stress management), along with conducive social and physical environment features (e.g., attractive local parks), are key to success.

INDIVIDUAL AND INTERPERSONAL MODELS

Individual-level models focus on personal factors that influence behavior (e.g., knowledge, attitudes, beliefs, motivation, experiences, and skills), whereas interpersonal-level theories acknowledge how other people affect our health behaviors. Social cognitive theory is a popular theory that addresses behavior at the interpersonal level. This section covers the origins and guiding principles of individual and interpersonal models.

Individual and Interpersonal Models
- Social Cognitive Theory
- Origins and Guiding Principles
  - Learning Theory
  - Decision-Making Theory
  - Behavioral Choice Theory
  - Relapse Prevention Model

Social Cognitive Theory

Social cognitive theory (Bandura, 1986, 1997, 2001) has been applied successfully to changing physical activity behavior. This theory proposes that behavior change is affected by interactions among the environment, personal factors, and attributes of the behavior itself, a concept that has been called *reciprocal determinism* (figure 3.1; Bandura, 1986). In other words, each of these three forces may affect or be affected by the other two. Furthermore, making physical activity a regular behavior can result from direct reinforcement. For example, you might praise clients who have stayed with their program for three months. A person may also adopt habitual physical activity behaviors resulting from observing the consequences that others experience. For instance, Mary may decide to dust off her stationary bike after a friend has described how biking has helped her feel less stressed and thereby parent her children more effectively, especially if this is an issue that is particularly relevant for Mary.

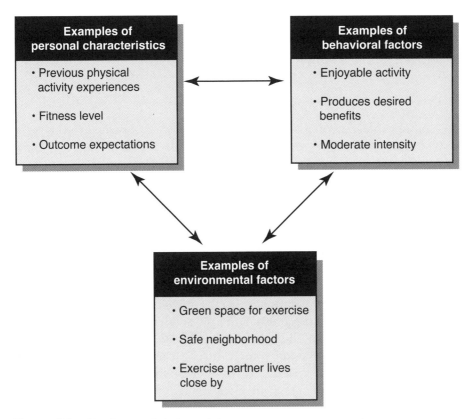

Figure 3.1 Reciprocal determinism.

A central concept in social cognitive theory is *self-efficacy*, or confidence in one's ability to successfully perform a particular behavior. People's perceptions that they can successfully perform a behavior increase the likelihood that they will engage in that behavior. Self-efficacy is behavior specific; for example, people may be confident that they can cut down their fat intake but not believe that they will stay physically active. To be even more specific, they may feel confident that they can maintain a walking program but not confident that they could get themselves to a gym four times a week for a fitness class. Self-efficacy has been shown to be related to physical activity behavior (Lewis et al., 2002; Sallis et al., 1989); therefore, it is important to evaluate and, if necessary, improve a client's self-efficacy for the type of activity you are targeting. Chapter 4 discusses measuring self-efficacy; the questionnaire for self-efficacy (questionnaire 4.2) can be adapted for a specific type of physical activity (e.g., walking). Included throughout part II are strategies for enhancing self-efficacy.

According to social cognitive theory, people must also believe that positive outcomes (*outcome expectations*) will follow if they are physically active and that these positive outcomes (e.g., weight maintenance, lower cholesterol) outweigh any negative outcomes they might also experience (e.g., physical discomfort during activity; Bandura, 1997). People must value these positive outcomes, whether they have short-term (e.g., feeling more energetic following physical activity) or long-term effects (e.g., warding off heart disease or diabetes).

Origins and Guiding Principles

Many popular interpersonal- and individual-level theories, such as the social cognitive theory and the transtheoretical model (discussed in chapter 2), have deep roots and incorporate constructs from learning, decision-making, and behavioral choice theories, along with cognitive behavioral therapy approaches (e.g., relapse prevention).

Learning Theory

Learning theories (Skinner, 1953) have also been widely applied to physical activity behavior change. According to learning theory, people are more likely to be physically active when the right circumstances are in place and pleasurable consequences occur because of physical activity (figure 3.2). For example, clients are more likely to be physically active when a place to exercise is readily available, they have time set aside, and they have already experienced a sense of accomplishment after squeezing in 30 minutes of activity on a previous day. In turn, if these clients find activity rewarding, they will be more likely to create the circumstances that will allow them to be active in the future.

Learning theory also acknowledges that when developing a new, complex behavior, such as physical activity, it is crucial to start with small steps and then progress slowly toward the desired result. This is called *shaping*. Often, newly physically active people start by setting goals that are too difficult, such as walking every day for 45 minutes. Likewise, program developers often set up programs that are too frequent, long, or intense for those who are newly

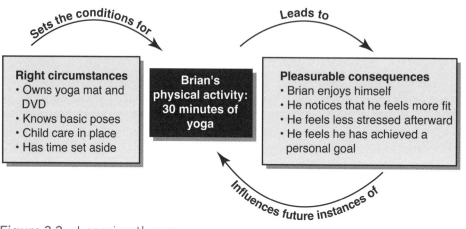

Figure 3.2 Learning theory.

physically active, such as three 60-minute kickboxing classes per week. As a result, the new exerciser becomes frustrated or injured and thus drops out before establishing the physical activity habit. However, by setting smaller, achievable goals (e.g., starting off with a 10-minute walk once a week, then gradually building to a 30-minute walk several times a week), the new exerciser can develop a sense of accomplishment and learn strategies for overcoming barriers that may have led to failure in the past.

By starting off with small goals (e.g., scheduling time, taking a walk even when tired, asking a family member to look after the kids for half an hour), your clients can take steps that are necessary for regular physical activity. As they become skilled at each of these small steps, the goal is then gradually increased (e.g., adding 5 minutes of daily activity each week). A reward can be planned for each goal that is achieved.

It is critical that your clients understand the importance of starting off slowly to avoid setting themselves up for failure and injury. For years people have been hearing "no pain, no gain," "feel the burn," and other messages that intense exercise in an all-or-none format is needed to gain benefits. We now know from the scientific literature that these extremes are unnecessary for health. However, if your clients do not understand that your approach is consistent with the newer recommendations and beneficial to their health, they may disregard your suggestions.

Learning theory also informs us that acquiring a new behavior typically requires frequent rewards and many pleasant consequences, at least in the beginning. This is particularly relevant to physical activity, which is often perceived as immediately punishing (e.g., time-consuming, painful, tiring), while many of its rewards (e.g., becoming healthier, feeling more energetic) do not occur for quite a while. Therefore, some programs have offered immediate incentives such as praise, social media reactions ("likes"), virtual awards (e.g., badges), or financial incentives for participation until natural reinforcers such as stress relief and muscle tone are achieved. Research supports the use of small, immediate (vs. larger, delayed) rewards. For example, Adams and colleagues found that as little as $1 per day increased physical activity, even among adults living at or above the median U.S. household income (Adams et al., 2017).

However, programs based on extrinsic rewards may not help people stay active over the long term (Glanz & Rimer, 1995). When a program that uses prizes to encourage participation or attendance ends, participants tend to go back to their sedentary lifestyles. Therefore, it is important to also incorporate strategies that enhance natural rewards from exercise (e.g., encouraging participants to set up their own support networks or helping them find activities they enjoy and can see themselves doing for a while) so participants will be more likely to keep exercising after your formal involvement is over.

Although it is important for people to eventually experience intrinsic rewards (e.g., a feeling of accomplishment, increased strength *and* or vigor),

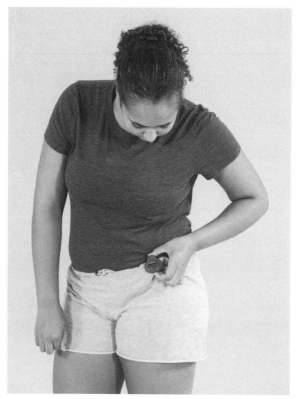
Pedometers can help remind you to add more steps to your day.

this can take quite some time, especially for clients who do not tend to use intrinsic rewards in other aspects of their lives. Reminders for physical activity can increase the likelihood that a person will become physically active. Pedometers and other wearable devices can serve as visual prompts to take more steps. Text messages, multimedia message services, and push notifications from smart phone applications have also been used to successfully remind individuals to be active.

Decision-Making Theory

Decision-making theory attempts to explain how people decide whether to engage in a particular behavior based on their comparison of the perceived benefits versus the perceived costs of the behavior (Janis & Mann, 1977). In other words, we are more likely to be active if we believe that the benefits of being active (e.g., improved health, stress relief) outweigh the costs (e.g., time taken away from other activities, getting hot and sweaty; figure 3.3). A person's weighing of the possible gains against the difficulties or losses experienced because of behavior change is often referred to as *decisional balance*.

People in the later stages of motivational readiness for change perceive more benefits of being physically active (e.g., more energy, less stress), whereas

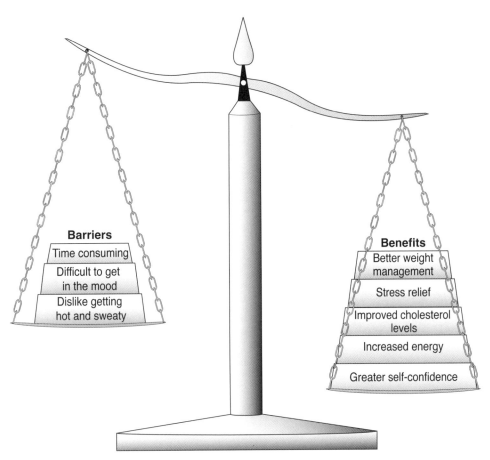

Figure 3.3 People are more likely to be motivated if they perceive that the benefits outweigh the barriers.

people in the earlier stages perceive more disadvantages (e.g., uncomfortable, too time-consuming) than advantages (Marcus, Rakowski, & Rossi, 1992). One way you might use this theory in a program is to have your clients write down what they think they will both gain and lose from participating in physical activity, both in the short and long term. You can then use this list to discuss anticipated barriers and ways to increase perceived benefits (Marcus, Rakowski, & Rossi, 1992; Wankel, 1984). In appendix A, we provide a simple measurement tool (questionnaire 4.4) you can use with clients to assess their decisional balance toward physical activity.

Behavioral Choice Theory

Behavioral choice theory is based on decision-making theory but also incorporates research in the areas of learning, planning, and economics (Epstein, 1998). This theory attempts to explain how people decide among the behavioral options available to them and how they then use their time among various activities, both sedentary and active. According to this theory, people have a choice between being sedentary and being physically active, and this choice is influenced by many factors, such as the availability of physical activities versus sedentary activities, perceived benefits versus barriers, reinforcement (i.e., rewards, both tangible and perceived), and degree of effort (figure 3.4). For example, reducing the accessibility of sedentary behaviors (e.g., parking spaces that are close to the building) and increasing the cost of being sedentary (e.g., a staircase close to the building's entrance but the elevator down the hall so that it takes more effort to take the elevator than the stairs) are both methods for reducing sedentary behaviors.

Whether clients perform a behavior and whether they enjoy it depends partly on the options available. For example, when your clients come home from a stressful day at work, they can plop down on the couch to watch TV, sit and talk to a friend on the phone, or go out for a brisk walk. If you and your clients can find an option that is both enjoyable and readily available, they may choose an active pursuit rather than a sedentary one without having to throw the TV out or put a lock on the phone! For example, you might encourage your clients to arrange to walk with a friend right after work as a way to relieve stress. You might encourage them to combine their favorite

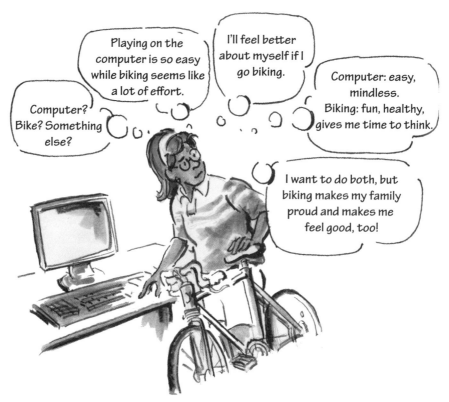

Figure 3.4 Behavioral choice theory.

sedentary activities with physical activity. For instance, if they enjoy watching television, you might encourage them to walk in place or on a treadmill during their favorite show. Video game enthusiasts could try switching to more active exergames, which have been shown to increase physical activity levels in numerous past studies with various populations (Street et al., 2017). In fact, even older adults reported substantial enjoyment and engagement in exergames, along with improved balance and cognitive function (Ismail et al., 2022).

Another important component of the behavioral choice theory is that for people to experience rewarding consequences because of physical activity, they need to believe that they are freely choosing to be active and are not being active only to please someone else. If people perceive that they are being forced to initiate an activity program rather than choosing on their own to become more active, they may not be motivated to change their lifestyles to more physically active ones. Discussing how your clients can benefit from physical activity or allowing them to set their own goals for physical activity rather than giving them the goal you think is best can help them recognize that the choice of becoming active is theirs.

Finally, choosing an active over a sedentary behavior depends in part on the time delay between making the choice and reaping the benefits from that choice. For physical activity, many of the benefits (e.g., less risk of developing heart disease) are delayed, whereas the benefits of being sedentary (e.g., having fun watching a movie on television) are immediate. Therefore, it is important to encourage your clients to look for immediate, but often overlooked, rewards of being active (e.g., feeling energized, the pleasure gained from doing something good for oneself, being a good role model to friends and family), and to keep in mind the long-term effects of sedentary behaviors that are often forgotten at the moment of choice.

Relapse Prevention Model

Although the relapse prevention model (figure 3.5) was originally developed to better understand people's difficulty with addictive behaviors such as smoking and drinking (Marlatt & Gordon, 1985), it also has been useful in understanding and intervening to increase physical activity. The appeal of the relapse prevention model is that it is especially geared toward maintaining change over the long term. This is particularly important for a behavior such as physical activity because most people do not maintain it, and continuing to be active over time is necessary to preserve its benefits. In fact, that is probably the biggest challenge in promoting physical activity—it does not do much good for people if they do not stick with it. A recent study conducted among Latina adults found that physical activity lapses (reporting <60 min/wk of physical activity after previously reporting 60+ min/wk of physical activity) were fairly common (probability of 18% after 1 month of starting to exercise) and increased over time (34% after 4 months; Larsen et al., 2021).

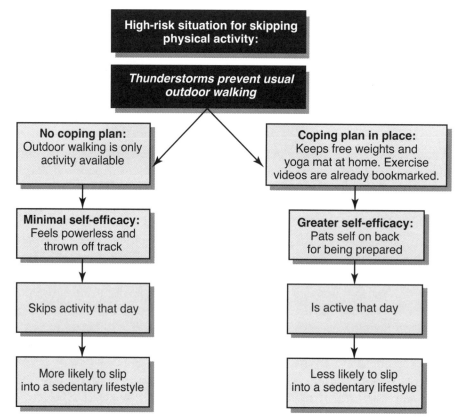

Figure 3.5 Diagram of the relapse prevention model.
Adapted from Marlatt and Gordon (1985).

Past work has also shown that men who were athletes in college but then stopped being active were no healthier than men who had never been active (Paffenbarger et al., 1986).

Programs based on the relapse prevention model help newly physically active people anticipate and plan for problems in continuing with their physical activity plans. Such problems include lack of time, social support, energy, motivation, skill, and/or facilities, as well as costs, inclement weather, and fear of injury (CDC 2022). This theory suggests that it is first important to identify situations that place people at high risk for not being physically active (e.g., putting in a lot of hours at work) and then to develop a game plan to avoid, or, if necessary, cope with, each of these situations (e.g., take two or three 10-minute walks as work breaks). If people find themselves in a situation in which they are at risk for not being active but use their skills to overcome the temptation to be sedentary, their self-efficacy is likely to increase. On the other hand, if they fail to be active, they are probably going to feel less confident in their abilities to handle similar situations in the future.

Another helpful aspect of the relapse prevention model is that it encourages people to distinguish between a *lapse* (e.g., a few days of not being physically active) and a *relapse* (e.g., an extended period of no physical activity) so that they do not fall prey to the *abstinence violation effect*. This term refers to people's tendency to give up altogether when they have slipped. For example, people who stop being active for a couple of weeks during a leisurely vacation may be disinclined to resume their activity program once they are home because they think, "What's the use? I'm out of the routine." By acknowledging such a break in the physical activity habit as a normal but temporary occurrence, they will be more likely to tell themselves, "Well, I had my break, but now it's time to start walking again." Inevitably, your clients will experience lapses, but these periods do not necessarily need to result in a return to a sedentary lifestyle. Your job is to help your clients plan for these potentially difficult situations.

CONCLUSION

You may have noticed that many of the ideas and program strategies discussed in this chapter are contained in the processes of change described in chapter 2. For example, the behavioral processes of rewarding yourself and committing yourself come from learning theory, social cognitive theory, and behavioral choice theory. The cognitive process of comprehending the benefits comes from behavioral choice theory, decision-making theory, and social cognitive theory. Increasing healthy opportunities directly relates to the environmental approach derived from the ecological model. The relapse prevention model relates to the processes of reminding yourself and substituting alternatives. Community models like CBPR and DOI emphasize the importance of enlisting social support and caring about consequences to others. Additionally, decisional balance, or the ratio of benefits to costs of physical activity (from decision-making theory), and self-efficacy (from social cognitive theory) have been shown to predict the stage of motivational readiness for physical activity (Marcus, Rakowski, & Rossi, 1992; Marcus, Selby, et al., 1992) and physical activity behavior (Lewis et al., 2002). These examples highlight the transtheoretical nature of the processes of change. We hope that, after reading this chapter, you also recognize that physical activity is not easily or completely described by any one theory or model. Table 3.3 illustrates how ideas from several theories can be translated into change strategies. In turn, these strategies can be combined to produce a comprehensive program that is likely to work. In other words, combining the approaches suggested by multiple theories is more likely to lead to success than depending on any one model alone.

Table 3.3 Promising Psychological Theories and Models for Promoting Physical Activity

Theory or model	Relevant ideas	Program strategies
Learning theory	Shaping Reinforcement Stimulus control Extrinsic vs. intrinsic rewards	Self-monitoring Goal setting Rewards Feedback
Decision-making theory	Perceived benefits Perceived barriers	Decisional balance sheet Removing barriers Problem-solving Enhancing benefits
Community models	Community-based participatory research principles Diffusion of innovations	Community engagement and outreach Collaborative partnerships with community Dissemination and implementation strategies
Behavioral choice theory	Reinforcement Benefits vs. barriers Perceived choice Availability of behavioral options	Rewards Decreasing sedentary options Including client in planning and decision-making Increasing options for activity
Social cognitive theory	Self-efficacy Outcome expectations Direct reinforcement Observational learning	Skill building Setting achievable goals Identifying benefits Tangible rewards Social support
Ecological model	Personal skills Institutional and community factors Physical environment Policies	Self-management Matching program to environmental opportunities Altering physical environments to include more activity options
Relapse prevention model	High-risk situations Self-efficacy Coping skills Abstinence violation effect	Planning Confidence building Problem-solving Identifying and changing negative thinking

More recent efforts to integrate the numerous theories of behavior change led to the development of the Behavior Change Wheel. At the foundation of this comprehensive model lie the main influences upon behavior change (Capability, Opportunity, Motivation; or COM-B) which are expanded into 14 subcategories (or domains) in the Theoretical Domains Framework and linked to the appropriate behavior change techniques for use with clients. For those interested in more detail on this topic, we recommend reading the "The Behaviour Change Wheel: A Guide to Designing Interventions" by Michie et al. (2014).

Overall, behavioral intervention research on physical activity is a relatively new area of scientific investigation, with very few studies conducted before 1990. Nonetheless, we have learned a great deal about physical activity behavior and how to help people become and stay more active. As a result, we can apply this knowledge to physical activity programs and make them more likely to succeed. Part II describes ways to implement the program strategies suggested by the models and theories described in this chapter within a stages of change framework.

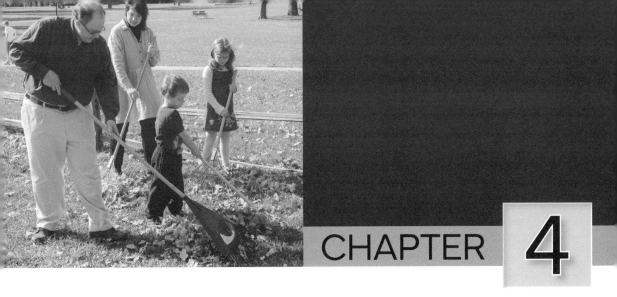

CHAPTER 4

Putting Theories to Work by Looking at Mediators of Change

Chapters 2 and 3 described some of the most promising psychological theories and models used to design successful physical activity programs. In this chapter we discuss constructs derived from these theories and models that are believed to produce, or *mediate*, behavior change. By becoming familiar with constructs derived from psychological and behavior change theories, you can incorporate strategies based on these constructs to build an effective physical activity program. We also include measures you can use to determine whether your intervention is affecting these constructs.

CONSIDER MEDIATORS OF PHYSICAL ACTIVITY BEHAVIOR CHANGE

When assessing the effectiveness of your interventions, you should consider not only measures of physical activity behavior but also changes in relevant psychological and behavioral mediators of physical activity behavior change. By paying attention to the parts of your program that were effective in helping your clients move toward a physically active lifestyle, you can learn what strategies work best for changing physical activity behaviors and get ideas for improving future programs (Baranowski et al., 1998; Bauman et al., 2002; Larsen et al., 2021; Linke et al., 2014). In other words, is your intervention successful for the reasons suggested by the theory you used to design it? For instance, if encouraging your client to track physical activity and set goals appears to be partly responsible for your client's increases in physical activity, then you probably will want to incorporate those strategies into a program you design for someone else.

Assessing psychosocial constructs related to change becomes especially important as we work to discover what helps unmotivated people move toward considering a more active lifestyle. For people in stage 1 (not thinking about change) or stage 2 (thinking about change), it is probably unrealistic to expect them to increase their actual activity to meet the national physical activity guidelines. Instead, a more realistic goal for these clients would be to promote change in factors that could lead to more physical activity down the road (e.g., identifying the pros of physical activity, enhanced self-efficacy). Helping less motivated people even start thinking about how their health and outlook might improve if they were to be more active should be considered a successful outcome. Therefore, learning what needs to happen within people for change to occur (i.e., discovering the mediators) is well worth your time and effort, as illustrated by the example Examining Mediators.

LEARNING HOW IT WORKS
Examining Mediators

This case example demonstrates the usefulness of looking at change in the theoretical constructs used to design a physical activity intervention. In this study, sedentary but healthy Latina women received Spanish-language printed materials on physical activity or other wellness topics (Marcus et al., 2013). The physical activity program was theoretically based and used constructs derived from social cognitive theory and the transtheoretical model. In this program participants received motivationally tailored manuals along with individualized feedback reports on their progress in self-reported physical activity, stage of motivational readiness, self-efficacy, and cognitive and behavioral processes of change. (The Seamos Saludables study is described in more detail in chapter 5.) The feedback reports were about four pages and provided each participant with information regarding any personal improvements or declines in these areas and their standing in comparison with others who had become active. These materials were sent via mail over six months, with four mailings in month one, two in months two to three, and one in months four to six.

The participants in the physical activity program reported significantly greater increases in physical activity compared to those who received the wellness materials at six months. The investigators were interested in looking at possible changes in the theoretical constructs used in the individually tailored intervention to learn what aspects of the intervention made it more effective than the wellness program. What they found was that participants who had received the individually tailored intervention had greater increases in social support for physical activity compared to the wellness control group from baseline to after treatment, and these increases in social support were responsible for the improvements in physical activity (Marquez et al., 2016).

Moreover, results indicated that different types of support may be important at varying time points. For example, help from family may get you started with physical activity, but supportive friends play more of a role in continuing these healthy habits. This analysis of possible mediating constructs can be used to develop more effective strategies in future programs.

The theoretical model that serves as the basis for a program suggests which factors might be responsible for producing change in physical activity behavior. For example, a program based on social cognitive theory may focus on improving self-efficacy and outcome expectations for physical activity because changes in these factors are thought to lead, in turn, to more physical activity. When you hypothesize about possible mediators of your program's success, keep in mind that several mediators may be working at once (Baranowski et al., 1998; Koring et al., 2012; Napolitano et al., 2008). For example, self-efficacy, outcome expectations, and the use of several behavior change processes may mediate the results of your intervention. Therefore, it is wise to consider and measure several possible mediators. Combining theories (e.g., the transtheoretical model and social cognitive theory) and building a program around several possible mediators (e.g., self-efficacy, enjoyment) are likely to make the program more successful, as shown in figure 4.1.

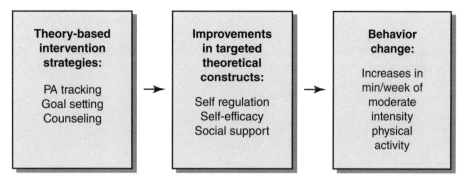

Figure 4.1 Using theoretical constructs to change physical activity motivation.

> ### *LEARNING HOW IT WORKS*
> #### Combining Theoretical Models and Targeting Multiple Mediators
>
> Why might you wish to target more than one theory or mediator when designing physical activity programs? There are many reasons. Health behaviors, such as physical activity, are complicated and multicomponent. Barriers and attitudes toward engaging in physical activity can vary among different groups. A single theory may serve in one setting, but in others, you may find it helpful to combine theories and pull constructs from different models to best address the specific factors involved in helping your clients adopt physical activity (and continue it).
>
> The Pasos Hacia la Salud study involved a web-based intervention that used theoretical constructs from both social cognitive theory and the stages of change theory to help 205 Latinas incorporate home-based moderate-to-vigorous intensity physical activity into their daily lives (Larsen et al., 2021). The women received individually tailored online feedback reports regarding their current stage of change for physical activity, self-efficacy, and cognitive and behavioral strategies. Social cognitive theory constructs were also targeted through physical activity coaching (on physical activity planning, goal setting, and social support), online tip sheets (on trying new activities, avoiding boredom), and resources (links to aerobic videos, walking route maps), because similar past studies found that participants who successfully adopted physical activity reported changes in these social cognitive theory variables. Results from this study supported the combined theoretical approach, because participants receiving the intervention reported increasing their physical activity by 50 more minutes per week at six months (31 more min/wk based on accelerometer recordings) than control group participants.
>
> This study also examined multiple mediators for how the intervention worked, which is reasonable because often not just one factor drives complex health behavior change. Many mechanisms could be expected to play a role in producing increases in physical activity. Accordingly, in the Pasos study, we hypothesized that the intervention worked by addressing the social cognitive theory and transtheoretical model constructs of self-efficacy, behavioral processes, cognitive processes, social support, and enjoyment, which in turn led to more minutes per week of physical activity. To test this hypothesis, we first examined physical activity and self-efficacy, behavioral processes, cognitive processes, and enjoyment at six months and found greater increases at six months among participants who received the intervention versus control. Next, we examined associations between changes in these variables and found that only changes in self-efficacy were associated with changes in self-reported and accelerometer-measured physical activity, whereas improvements in other variables (social support

from friends and enjoyment, cognitive and behavioral processes) were associated with just one or the other (self-reported or measured physical activity, respectively). Finally, self-efficacy emerged as a mediator for both self-reported and measured physical activity, with enjoyment mediating the intervention effects on self-reported physical activity (Larsen et al., 2021). Such findings emphasize the importance of considering multiple mediators from more than one theory (e.g., self-efficacy and enjoyment) when designing strategies for your physical activity program.

FACTORS THAT ENHANCE PHYSICAL ACTIVITY

In this section we describe some constructs derived from psychological theories and models that are believed to create change in physical activity behavior. As you will see, social cognitive theory and the transtheoretical model are the most commonly used theoretical frameworks in studies of physical activity mediators (Lewis et al., 2002; Rhodes & Pfaeffli, 2010; Rhodes et al., 2021).

Cognitive and Behavioral Processes of Change

According to the Transtheoretical model, people use various cognitive and behavioral strategies and techniques to progress through the stages of motivational readiness for change (DiClemente et al., 1991; Prochaska & DiClemente, 1983). People in the later stages tend to use more of these processes than people in the earlier stages (Bernard et al., 2014; Marcus, Rossi, et al., 1992). Numerous studies have shown increased use of behavioral processes to be significantly related to increases in physical activity behavior (Dunn et al., 1997; Lewis et al., 2002; Lewis et al., 2006; Nichols et al., 2000; Papandonatos et al., 2012; Pinto et al., 2001; Sallis et al., 1999), whereas the findings on cognitive processes serving as mediators of physical activity have been mixed. Cognitive processes may be particularly important for helping people in the earlier stages of motivational readiness move toward changing their actual physical activity behavior (Marcus, Rossi, et al., 1992; Rosen, 2000). More recent results have indicated that both cognitive and behavioral processes are used to progress through the stages of change (Bernard et al., 2014; Dishman et al., 2010; Kanning, 2010; Marcus, Selby, et al., 1992; Rhodes et al., 2021). Examples of each of these processes of change are found in chapter 2.

Measuring Processes of Change

A client's use of the processes of change for physical activity behavior can be measured with questionnaire 4.1 in appendix A, which we and our colleagues developed (Marcus, Rossi, et al., 1992). This questionnaire has been used in many physical activity studies. When people's scores on these items increase, it is usually a good indicator that they are becoming more active (Dunn et al., 1997). The processes of change are the strategies and techniques people use to change their thinking and their behavior; your clients are therefore likely to increase their use of many of the processes of change long before they are meeting national guidelines for a physically active lifestyle.

You may want to have clients complete this questionnaire every three months so that you can learn whether they are making progress toward behavior change even if they are not meeting their specific physical activity goals. Recall that the stage of motivation for change when clients first come to see you has a great impact on how quickly they increase their use of the processes of change. The setting in which you work might also affect which processes of change increase first and how quickly clients put them to use. For example, if you are a personal trainer at a gym, you are more likely to start working with clients on behavior change, and thus you are more likely to see increases in the behavioral processes of change. However, if you work at a community center (e.g., YMCA), you may see changes in your clients' cognitive processes before changes in their behavioral processes. Most published studies indicate that it is important for people to first increase their use of cognitive processes and then of behavioral processes. However, some studies indicate that the order is not important; people need to increase their use of all (or most) of the processes of change to become and stay regularly active (Marcus, Rossi, et al., 1992).

For each process of change, the average score can range from one to five. Table 4.1 shows typical scores for the four items in each process group for people in each stage of motivational readiness for change. Use this as a guide for understanding where your clients are in the change process and on which areas to focus to help them start and continue a program of regular physical activity. If the survey results are similar on a number of processes, you can choose either a single process or, in collaboration with your client, several processes to work on.

Table 4.1 Average Scores by Stage for the Processes of Change Questionnaire

Process	Stage 1	Stage 2	Stage 3	Stage 4	Stage 5
Increasing knowledge	1.88	2.57	2.76	3.11	2.99
Being aware of risks	1.92	2.41	2.26	2.72	2.46
Caring about consequences to others	1.82	2.43	2.46	2.74	2.47
Comprehending benefits	2.14	3.13	3.22	3.66	3.28

	Stage				
Increasing healthy opportunities	2.14	2.55	2.75	2.81	2.79
Substituting alternatives	1.71	2.24	2.72	3.35	3.55
Enlisting social support	1.78	2.25	2.42	2.80	2.64
Rewarding oneself	1.52	2.25	2.54	2.99	3.01
Committing oneself	2.08	2.94	3.17	3.83	3.68
Reminding oneself	1.42	1.85	2.02	2.30	2.20

Scoring Processes of Change

For each process, average the individual items by adding each group (shown in table 4.2) together and dividing by four. Do not score an individual process if fewer than three items were answered.

Table 4.2 Grouping Related Items on the Processes of Change Questionnaire

Process	Items
Increasing knowledge	5, 8, 17, 28
Being aware of risks	11, 12, 13, 14
Caring about consequences to others	30, 33, 34, 37
Comprehending benefits	15, 31, 35, 38
Increasing healthy opportunities	10, 22, 32, 36
Substituting alternatives	1, 21, 39, 40
Enlisting social support	16, 19, 24, 25
Rewarding oneself	7, 18, 20, 23
Committing oneself	2, 4, 6, 27
Reminding oneself	3, 9, 26, 29

Self-Efficacy

Self-efficacy refers to confidence in one's ability to perform specific behaviors in specific situations (Bandura, 1986, 1997). For example, in many parts of the United States, people often have higher self-efficacy (i.e., feel very self-confident) regarding their ability to maintain a walking program during the spring and summer months but do not see themselves keeping up with their activity in the cold, snowy winter. This is not surprising, given that maintaining some type of physical activity in the winter often requires a new set of behaviors, such as going to an indoor facility or learning how to dress appropriately for activity in cold weather. Another example illustrates how self-efficacy is also behavior specific. Many people have a high level of self-efficacy for some types of physical activity, such as brisk walking, but feel less confident in their ability to incorporate additional types of activity (e.g., muscle strengthening activities) that would be beneficial for increasing variety and reducing the risks of boredom and overuse injuries. Some studies have investigated self-efficacy for physical activity across various situations, such as during vacation, when injured, and during bad weather (Marcus, Selby, et al., 1992; Mendoza-Vasconez et al., 2018). Others have looked at self-efficacy for various components of being physically active, such as making time for and continuing with activity (Frerichs et al., 2020; Sallis et al., 1988).

According to social cognitive theory, self-efficacy is the most important mediator of behavior change (Bandura, 1986, 1997), and this has been demonstrated across studies looking at mediating constructs of successful interventions (Brassington et al., 2002; Lewis et al., 2002; Teixeira et al., 2015). In other words, improved self-efficacy leads to higher levels of physical activity at some later time (usually measured three to six months after the start of the program). These findings have been corroborated by web-based physical activity interventions among Latinas and women with a family history of breast cancer, in which self-efficacy mediated intervention effects on moderate-to-vigorous physical activity (Larsen et al., 2021; Marinac et al., 2018).

Measuring Self-Efficacy

We recommend measuring physical activity–specific self-efficacy with questionnaire 4.2 in appendix A, which we and our colleagues developed (Marcus, Selby, et al., 1992). This brief, five-item questionnaire measures the major components of self-efficacy and has been used in many physical activity studies. Previous studies have confirmed the scale's reliability and validity among different populations (e.g., adults and college students living in the United States, Australia, and Finland; Cardinal et al., 2003; Marcus & Owen, 1992; Marcus et al., 1994; Mendoza-Vasconez et al., 2018). Moreover, if time is an issue, a study among Spanish-speaking Latinas found that collapsing the five response options into three (Not Confident, Slightly Confident/Moderately Confident, Very Confident/Extremely Confident) may reduce burden and improve precision of the scale (Mendoza-Vasconez et al., 2018). People's self-efficacy scores almost always increase as they become more active. As with the processes of change questionnaire, we encourage you to administer the self-efficacy questionnaire to your clients every three months. If clients' scores on this measure are not increasing, this is a red flag; you need to discuss this lack of self-efficacy with them because their belief that they cannot succeed with physical activity does not bode well for their becoming and staying active for life.

Scoring Self-Efficacy

Calculate the score on the self-efficacy questionnaire by computing the average of all five items for each client. If any item is unanswered, have the client fill it in before scoring. A higher score on this measure indicates greater self-efficacy. Increased self-efficacy is important for a person to adopt and maintain a program of regular physical activity.

Exercise Goals and Plans

Goal setting and planning are self-regulation skills that play a major role in the successful initiation and maintenance of behavior change (Rovniak et al., 2002). Because lack of time is a common physical activity barrier, people often find it helpful to review their calendars and schedule their physical activity sessions in advance. Exercise planning allows clients to think through the logistics and coordinate with others (e.g., exercise partners, child-care providers). It also builds commitment; walks booked in advance are more likely to happen. Howlett and colleagues (2019) found that goal setting was the most frequently used physical activity behavior change strategy, which is unsurprising because setting exercise goals can keep clients motivated and build confidence. Together, planning and goal setting provide direction and structure for achieving a more active lifestyle. Higher levels of self-regulatory skills (e.g., goal setting and planning) have been associated with regular exercise in past studies (with college students and older adults with MS; Baird et al., 2021; Rovniak et al., 2002). Moreover, these constructs emerged as mediators of physical activity behavior change among diverse samples (e.g., postnatal women, adolescent girls, older Japanese adults; Fjeldsoe et al., 2013; Harada, 2022; Taymoori & Revalds Lubans, 2008).

Measuring Exercise Goals and Plans

We recommend measuring exercise with goal setting and planning questionnaires. Dr. Rovniak and colleagues (2002) developed two brief, 10-item self-regulation questionnaires that have been used in many physical activity studies and have demonstrated good internal consistency and stability over time.

Scoring Exercise Goals and Planning

To calculate the scores for exercise goals and planning, first reverse score planning items two, three, and seven, and then compute the average of all 10 items for each scale.

Social Support

Social support is believed to be another strong mediator of behavior change (Lewis et al., 2002; Marquez et al., 2016; Sarason & Sarason, 1985). The four types of social support are instrumental, informational, emotional, and appraising (Cohen et al., 1985).

- *Instrumental* support involves giving another person something tangible to encourage behavior change. Examples of instrumental support are giving someone a ride to a yoga class or letting them borrow your bicycle.

- *Informational* social support involves helping a person make behavior changes by providing relevant information. For example, you might tell a friend about an upcoming fun run or talk to your sibling about the strategies you use to keep yourself motivated.

- *Emotional* support is letting other people know that you care about them and how they are doing in their attempt to change their behavior. When you call friends or family members to see how they are faring with their attempt to walk 20 minutes each day, you are offering emotional support.

- *Appraising* involves providing feedback and encouragement to someone learning a new physical activity skill. Aerobics instructors provide this type of support when they tell class participants that they have noticed their improvement over the last few weeks. Physical activity tips and advice are often shared via social media channels (e.g., Facebook discussion groups), where participants can provide feedback and comment on each other's photos and posts.

There is evidence that both the type and source of social support for physical activity matter. Data from the British Whitehall II study indicated that emotional and practical support from a client's closest person can help with active lifestyle maintenance (Kouvonen et al., 2012). As illustrated in the earlier examples, social support can come from many sources (e.g., family members, friends, coworkers, exercise instructors, online communities, and mobile applications; Miller et al., 2002; Stoddard et al., 2004; USDHHS, 1996; Yang et al., 2015). Some sources may be more important than others, depending on the situation. A systematic review found a strong relationship between physical activity and social support from family but not from friends for older adults (Smith et al., 2017).

Physical activity research has looked at both general social support and social support specific to physical activity. Studies comparing the two found that they are quite distinct (Sallis et al., 1987; Smith et al., 2017). People may believe that they have good social support in most areas of their lives (e.g., a spouse who shares household responsibilities, friends and family members with whom they feel comfortable sharing their feelings and concerns), yet they may believe that few people share their interest in physical activity, can give advice about being physically active, or will help with child-care responsibilities so that they can make the time for physical activity. In a program designed to help sedentary mothers of young children increase their physical activity, increased support from the children's fathers was associated with the mothers' ability to become more physically active (Miller et al., 2006).

Measuring Social Support for Physical Activity

We recommend using a questionnaire that was developed specifically to measure physical activity–related social support from family and friends (questionnaire 4.3 in appendix A; Sallis et al., 1987).

The client should answer each question for both family and friends (there is a separate column to check for each). This instrument asks about exercise-related support obtained in the last three months, so you may want to administer it at three-month intervals to detect any changes. If your client receives a low score for social support from either friends or family, you may want to suggest some strategies for enhancing social support (e.g., sign up for group walks, join a hiking club) because higher social support has been associated with greater success in changing health habits and with better physical activity adherence in adult and adolescent populations (Courneya & McAuley, 1995; Mendonça et al., 2014; Miller et al., 2002; Monteiro et al., 2021; Oka et al., 1995; Rodrigues et al., 2023; Sallis et al., 1987).

Scoring Social Support for Physical Activity

To score the measure for social support for physical activity, first invert the responses to questions seven and eight (1 = 5, 2 = 4, 3 = 3, 4 = 2, 5 = 1). Then add all the items for family support and all the items for friend support separately. Higher scores reflect more perceived social support from these people.

Decisional Balance

Decisional balance—the ratio of perceived benefits to barriers of change—comes from Janis and Mann's (1977) decision-making theory. Regarding physical activity behavior change, *decisional balance* refers to a person's perception of the benefits of physical activity compared to the negative aspects (Janis & Mann, 1977; Marcus, Rakowski, et al., 1992). Some people view physical activity in a positive light, whereas others focus more on the downsides. Some perceived barriers are environmental, such as bad weather, an unsafe neighborhood for walking, and a lack of available parks, sidewalks, and bicycle paths. Other barriers are more personal, such as believing you do not have enough time or energy to be physically active after work. Fear of becoming injured, lack of motivation, and unhelpful friends or family members are other examples of personal barriers.

Decisional balance has been associated with physical activity behaviors in several studies (Abbaspour et al., 2017; Bradley et al., 2015; Jiménez-Zazo et al., 2020). Differences in decisional balance tend to correspond to the various stages of motivational readiness. People in stage one (not thinking about change) perceive more barriers than benefits to change, whereas those in the later stages perceive more benefits than barriers (Abbaspour et al., 2017; Bradley et al., 2015; Jiménez-Zazo et al., 2020; Marcus & Owen, 1992; Marcus, Rakowski, et al., 1992).

Research has shown that for people to become more active, they need to see many benefits and few barriers to becoming more active. Over time, people tend to see more benefits than barriers to physical activity, which is important to keeping them active over the long term. Indeed, higher scores on the decisional balance measure (i.e., viewing physical activity in a more positive than negative light) have been shown to predict increases in physical activity behavior (Dunn et al., 1997; Pinto et al., 2001). Interestingly, decisional balance may be more or less relevant when working with different populations. For example, in focus groups, Latinas indicated that the construct did not resonate with them as an important factor in adopting physical activity (Pekmezi et al., 2009). Accordingly, the measure has not been included in several recent studies with this population.

Measuring Decisional Balance

We recommend using the decisional balance questionnaire (questionnaire 4.4 in appendix A) that we and our colleagues developed (Marcus, Rakowski, et al., 1992) to measure physical activity decision-making. This questionnaire measures a client's perceived benefits of and barriers to physical activity.

Scoring Decisional Balance

Compute the averages of the 10 pro items and the 6 con items.

- Pros = (item 1 + item 2 + item 4 + item 5 + item 6 + item 8 + item 9 + item 10 + item 12 + item 14) / 10
- Cons = (item 3 + item 7 + item 11 + item 13 + item 15 + item 16) / 6

The difference in the averages (i.e., pros minus cons) is the decisional balance score. Decisional balance scores greater than zero indicate that your client sees more benefits than barriers to being active. The larger the score, the more benefits your client sees relative to the barriers. A score less than zero indicates that your client sees more barriers than benefits to being physically active. The larger the negative score, the more barriers your client sees relative to benefits. It is important to help your client see both more benefits and fewer barriers to physical activity. If your program is successful, you will likely see scores on this questionnaire move from negative to positive and then continue to rise.

Outcome Expectations

The term *outcome expectations* refers to the value people place on the outcomes or consequences they believe will occur because of being physically active. These outcomes can be positive or negative. Some may occur immediately after being active (e.g., feeling energized), whereas other outcomes require being physically active for some time (e.g., losing weight or having more muscle tone). Researchers have found associations between outcome expectations and physical activity (Chu & Wang, 2022; Morrison & Stuifbergen, 2014; Williams et al., 2005). In fact, some studies have found that people with higher outcome expectations for exercise were more likely to adopt and maintain regular physical activity (Brassington et al., 2002; Crozier & Spink, 2017; Hallam & Petosa, 1998; McFadden et al., 2022; Williams et al., 2005). While positive outcome expectations, such as health benefits, improved body image, and stress reduction, have been shown to predict physical activity behavior, the relationship between positive outcome expectations and physical activity may be stronger among older adults than younger individuals. Small associations have also been found between negative outcome expectations and physical activity, with personal barriers (e.g., costs, work conflicts, and fatigue) predicting lower levels of physical activity (Williams et al., 2005).

Measuring Outcome Expectations

The brief Outcome Expectations for Exercise scale (Resnick et al., 2000) can be used to measure your clients' expected benefits from activity (see questionnaire 4.5 in appendix A). This scale asks about both the physical and mental benefits expected. If you find that your clients have low expectations for physical activity, you should work with them to identify some benefits they are likely to experience because of their activity. Doing so may help strengthen their outcome expectations, which in turn may improve their physical activity behavior.

Scoring Outcome Expectations

This measure is scored by adding the ratings for all the items and dividing by nine to get the average of all nine items. Scores can range from one to five, with one indicating low outcome expectations for exercise and five suggesting high outcome expectations. Although the measure is used to obtain an overall score for outcome expectations, you can look at your clients' scores on the individual items to determine the areas in which they believe they are less likely to benefit. Then you can focus on improving these areas.

Enjoyment

People who say they enjoy physical activity tend to be those who become and stay active (Wankel, 1993). Indeed, enjoyment of physical activity is associated with stage of motivational readiness for change, adherence to structured exercise programs, and increased levels of physical activity behavior (Klompstra et al., 2022; Leslie et al., 1999; Lewis et al., 2016; Rovniak et al., 2002; Stevens et al., 2000; USDHHS, 1996; Williams et al., 2006). A recent study found that physical activity enjoyment completely mediated the relationship between exercise motivation and physical activity among heart failure patients (Klompstra et al., 2022). Thus, consider focusing on enhancing enjoyment early on, because even the most motivated clients may struggle to continue physical activity if they do not enjoy it. Enjoyment of physical activity is not directly related to any specific theory, yet some have argued that it can be conceptualized as a type of outcome expectancy because enjoyment has been assumed to be related to a person's willingness to be active (Williams et al., 2005). Therefore, if we can help a client enjoy physical activity, the client is more likely to be active later. This is supported by a study that found that a school-based intervention enhanced adolescent girls' enjoyment of physical activity, which in turn led to increased physical activity behavior (Dishman et al., 2005).

Measuring Physical Activity Enjoyment

The Physical Activity Enjoyment Scale (see questionnaire 4.6 in appendix A) is an 18-item measure that can be used to determine how enjoyable your client finds exercise. The developers of this measure say that it can be used for any physical activity (Kendzierski & DeCarlo, 1991). You can help clients who score low on this measure find activities that are more pleasurable, or you can adjust their activities, so they are less unpleasant (e.g., suggest they listen to music while being active, engage in a moderate-intensity activity rather than a vigorous one, or talk to a partner during activity).

Scoring Physical Activity Enjoyment

For items 1, 4, 5, 7, 9, 10, 11, 13, 14, 16, and 17, assign point values as follows:

If the client answered
- 1, give a score of 7
- 2, give a score of 6
- 3, give a score of 5
- 4, give a score of 4
- 5, give a score of 3
- 6, give a score of 2
- 7, give a score of 1

Then add all the items. Higher scores reflect greater enjoyment of physical activity. You can give this measure to your clients periodically (e.g., every month or two) to see whether their enjoyment increases as they become more skilled and physically fit over time. Or you can have your clients complete this questionnaire after you have made some suggestions for making physical activity more fun and they have had a chance to try your ideas. This can be a way of determining what makes activity more pleasurable for your client.

UNLOCK THE BLACK BOX

Although many physical activity programs are based on psychological theories and models, few studies test to see whether the program changed the theoretical constructs used to design the program (Baranowski et al., 1998; Lewis et al., 2002; Rhodes et al., 2021). To do this, researchers first must determine whether the program changed possible mediators. For example, did a program based on social cognitive theory, which emphasizes self-efficacy, really help participants become more confident in their ability to become and stay active, and did a change in self-efficacy lead to participants' actually becoming more physically active? Furthermore, interventions are more or less effective depending on the population. These concepts are explained in more detail in the sidebar, Learning How It Works.

LEARNING HOW IT WORKS
Moderators Versus Mediators

If you are interested in learning more about testing the theories you use to design your intervention, you should understand what is meant by the terms *mediator* and *moderator*. Although the terms are often used interchangeably in the literature, the function of a moderator is quite different from that of a mediator (Baron & Kenny, 1986; Bauman et al., 2002).

Moderators: A moderator is a factor used to divide participants into subgroups for whom the intervention works differently (Baron & Kenny, 1986; Bauman et al., 2002). Sometimes factors such as age, gender, health status, mood, and socioeconomic status may be related to the effectiveness of a program and therefore may serve as moderators.

For example, one study found that culturally and linguistically adapted theory-based physical activity interventions for Spanish-speaking Latinas were more effective for women with lower body mass indexes (BMIs) than women with higher BMIs (Hartman et al., 2011). In fact, participants with lower BMIs (e.g., 25 kg/m^2) reported on average 27.5 more minutes per week of activity at six months compared to those with higher BMIs (e.g., 30 kg/m^2). In this case BMI was a moderator of the intervention's effectiveness. Aspects of participants' physical environment (e.g., crime rate, availability of sidewalks, green space, and level of traffic congestion) may also serve as moderators that determine subgroups for whom a given intervention may be more or less effective (King et al., 2002). Moderators tell us *who* will benefit most from a program, but they do not tell us *how* the intervention

(continued)

Moderators Versus Mediators *(continued)*

works. To determine this, we look at factors that change because of a program: the mediators.

Mediators: In contrast to many moderators (e.g., age, gender), a mediator is always a factor that can help a given client change. A mediator represents the mechanism by which the intervention is believed to influence physical activity behavior (Baron & Kenny, 1986; Bauman et al., 2002). For example, you might design a program based on the social cognitive theory that attempts to help clients set goals and make plans for becoming active. The theory assumes that physical activity planning and goal setting will help your client become and stay physically active.

In this example, physical activity planning and goal setting are believed to be mediators of behavior change. For instance, prior to starting your program, you measure physical activity planning and goal setting and find that your clients are not making many physical activity plans or goals. After you complete your intervention and find that your clients have become more active, you decide to measure their physical activity planning and goal setting again. If you find that your clients now plan their physical activity and set goals, you have some evidence that your intervention's ability to improve physical activity goal setting and planning helped your clients become more active.

At a higher level of sophistication, you might track changes in physical activity planning and goal setting through repeated measurement of these variables to see whether changes occur first in these mediators prior to increases in physical activity behavior. If so, you will have demonstrated that changes in mediating variables in turn led to increases in physical activity. To learn more about various influences on physical activity, refer to Bauman and colleagues (2002) and Rhodes and colleagues (2017), and for a review of psychosocial mediators tested in various interventions, refer to Lewis and colleagues (2002) and Rhodes and colleagues (2021).

CONCLUSION

In this chapter we reviewed potential mediators of physical activity interventions. What is a mediator? Mediators are how people change (e.g., the strategies they use to increase physical activity). Constructs from the transtheoretical model and social cognitive theory have been shown to mediate physical activity change. In other words, increases in physical activity are often achieved through improvements in processes of change, self-efficacy, planning, goal setting, social support, decisional balance, outcome expectations, and enjoyment of physical activity. We defined and provided valid, reliable measures for each of these constructs, along with guidance on scoring the responses and interpreting the results. We also discussed how these potential mediators could be targeted for behavior change. Could including a client's family and friends in the program help that client be more active? Considering factors such as these, addressing them in your program, and then measuring them to see whether they change because of your program can help open up the "black box" of changing physical activity behavior. We also discussed the difference between mediators (how the physical activity intervention works) and moderators (for whom the intervention works). The chapters in part II discuss strategies for influencing physical activity mediators in further detail.

CHAPTER 5

Using the Stages Model for Successful Physical Activity Interventions

Much of our population is sedentary (over 25%, according to a 2022 Centers for Disease Control report), and most people who start an exercise program do not continue it over the long term (Dishman, 1994; Kahlert, 2015; Marcus et al., 2000; McEwan et al., 2022). Perhaps this is because many programs take a "one size fits all" approach that assumes clients are ready to be active.

The stages of motivational readiness for change model is founded on the idea that people differ in their levels of readiness to change their behavior. Therefore, programs need to use differing strategies and techniques to bring about desired behavior changes. For example, the program goal for a client starting in stage 1 (not thinking about change) could be to help the client begin to think about change by reading articles about the health, body image, and self-esteem benefits of physical activity. In contrast, the goal of a program for a client in stage 3 (doing some physical activity) might be using social support (e.g., walking partners) to build up to national physical activity guidelines.

In this chapter we describe a few physical activity programs that have used the stages of change model. Earlier programs could attract people who were already physically active but had a harder time reaching those who were not. Part of the reason for this may have been the program names; a program called Get Fit recruited people who were already active and wanted to become more fit or maintain their fitness. Programs targeted at people in stage 2 have used names such as Jump Start to Health.

JUMP START TO HEALTH: A WORKPLACE-BASED STUDY

The Jump Start to Health study examined the usefulness of a stage-matched physical activity program in the workplace for healthy, sedentary employees (Marcus, Emmons, et al., 1998). People in the stage-matched group received manuals specifically tailored to their stage of motivational readiness for change. The manual for those in stage 1 (not thinking about change), titled *Do I Need This?*, focused on increasing awareness of the benefits of activity and the barriers that prevent people from being active. This manual did not provide specific suggestions for starting an exercise routine. The manual for those thinking about change (stage 2), titled *Try It, You'll Like It*, included a

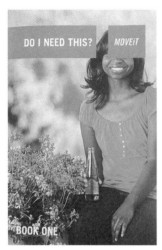
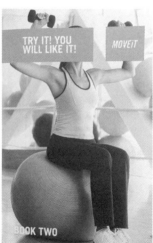
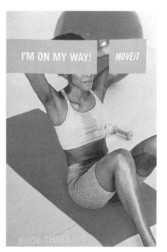
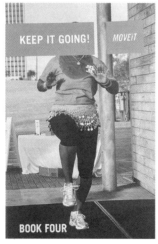
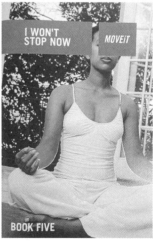

Manuals tailored to the various stages of motivational readiness for physical activity behavior change.

Dori Pekmezi

discussion of the reasons to stay inactive versus the reasons to become more active, learning to reward oneself, and setting realistic goals.

For those in stage 3 (doing some physical activity), *I'm on My Way* reviewed the benefits of activity, goal setting, and tips on safe and enjoyable activities and addressed obstacles to regular activity (e.g., lack of time, feeling too tired). *Keep It Going* provided information for those in stage 4 (doing enough physical activity) on the benefits of regular activity, staying motivated, rewarding oneself, enhancing confidence about being active, and overcoming obstacles. For those in stage 5 (making physical activity a habit), *I Won't Stop Now* emphasized the benefits of regular activity, avoiding injuries, setting goals, varying activities, rewarding oneself, and planning ahead.

An examination of participants' responses to questionnaires at the beginning of the program and three months later revealed that more participants who received stage-matched manuals reported becoming more active (37% vs. 27%) than those who received American Heart Association manuals (AHA, 1984a, 1984b, 1984c, 1984d, 1989). The stage-matched approach was particularly effective for those who entered the program in stages 1, 2, or 3, which is noteworthy because these are the people who are most likely to be your clients.

JUMP START: A COMMUNITY-BASED STUDY

In this community-based study, individually tailored physical activity feedback reports were developed and provided in addition to the previously mentioned stage-matched manuals. (Marcus, Bock, et al., 1998). The goal was to give participants tailored comparisons between their own behaviors and those of other participants who had been successful. Additionally, feedback informed participants about how they had changed since the last time they filled out the questionnaires so that they understood whether they were moving forward, sliding backward, or doing about the same on a variety of strategies and techniques shown to be important for becoming long-term physically active people.

Following are examples of two types of such feedback. The first example gives a comparison between the individual and other successful participants:

> *Your answers show that you are well aware of the benefits of regular exercise. This is something that you have in common with others in the program who have also made good progress. Because you already do some exercise, it's now important for you to gradually become more active and make exercise a more frequent and consistent part of your life. Now is the time to think about the things that could stop you from exercising regularly. Being prepared for the problems you may encounter is a big help in adhering to an exercise program. You will be better prepared to overcome obstacles by thinking about the kinds of thoughts and activities that will help you remain active during difficult periods.*

This is an example of feedback regarding the individual's change since the prior assessment:

Your answers show that since we last heard from you, you have been taking more responsibility for your own health and well-being. You are also becoming more aware of the importance of believing in yourself and your ability to remain active. That's great! However, you are thinking a bit less about these issues than others who have succeeded in becoming and staying active.

To make more progress, try making a commitment to being more active. Think about the things you have done before, achievements you have made, goals you have reached. Try setting small goals for yourself that you know you can meet, such as going for a short walk or adding a few extra minutes of activity into each day. This will help you strengthen your sense of accomplishment.

The individualized feedback concerned the topics of motivation, cognitive and behavioral strategies for becoming more active, barriers to and benefits from exercise, self-efficacy, and minutes of physical activity per week. Participants received printed reports and stage-matched manuals at the beginning of the program when they were first assessed by questionnaire and one, three, and six months later.

Results showed that those who received the individualized program were more likely to achieve recommended levels of physical activity (accumulating at least 30 minutes of physical activity/day at least 5 days/wk) and were more likely to maintain that activity through a 12-month follow-up period than were participants who were given standard materials promoting physical activity (Bock et al., 2001; Marcus, Bock, et al., 1998). Thus, this study shows that using materials matched to each participant's specific characteristics is helpful in increasing physical activity.

LEARNING HOW IT WORKS
Applying the Stages of Change Theory to Physical Activity Promotion in Underserved Populations

Given the success of these stage-matched manuals and individually tailored feedback reports among mostly non–Hispanic White participants in Jump Start, we began to explore how similar approaches could be used to address physical activity-related health disparities in underserved populations. When considering extending a program developed in one community to another, often changes must be made. This is best done in consultation and collaboration with the population of interest. We describe our prior efforts to adapt the individually tailored physical activity print intervention for use among Latinas in this section.

In the Seamos Activas study, the intervention materials and research measures were translated into Spanish through an iterative translation and back-translation process (Pekmezi et al., 2009). Twenty-five cognitive interviews were conducted with Latinas to improve the clarity of the intervention and assessment text and ensure that key messages were not lost in translation. For example, participants noted differences between the terms *exercise* and *physical activity*, with *exercise* more accurately conveying purposeful moderate-intensity activity. "Rewarding yourself for meeting exercise goals" had a materialistic connotation, compared to "doing something good for yourself." Changes were made to the intervention and assessment materials based on these findings (e.g., consistently referenced *exercise* in measures and materials). Six focus groups also identified culture-specific attitudes and barriers to physical activity for Latinas. Themes from participant feedback were incorporated into the intervention text and included balancing caregiver and household responsibilities, cultural norms about self-sacrifice, social support, partner negotiation, and dealing with inclement weather and neighborhood safety.

A small pilot randomized control trial (n = 93) found that the resulting culturally and linguistically adapted intervention for Latinas produced larger increases in moderate-intensity (or greater) physical activity from baseline (M = 16.56 min/wk, SD = 25.76) to six months (M = 147.27, SD = 241.55) than a wellness contact control arm (M = 11.88 min/wk, SD = 21.99 at baseline; M = 96.79, SD = 118.49 at 6 months), as well as significantly greater increases in cognitive and behavioral processes of change and available physical activity supplies and equipment at home (see health study manual pictures earlier in this chapter). Promising results were also found when adapting the individually tailored print intervention for use among African American women in the Deep South using similar processes (Pekmezi et al., 2016, 2017, 2020). Thus, while modifications will likely be necessary, successful theory-based programs developed in one community can be extended to another with great effect. Engaging the target population in this adaptation process is critical and will likely improve outcomes.

PROJECT ACTIVE: A COMMUNITY-BASED STUDY

Project Active also was based on the stages of motivational readiness for change model (Dunn et al., 1999). This two-year study compared a lifestyle physical activity program (which encouraged participants to fit in 10-minute walks whenever they could) with a structured exercise program (which offered free membership at a beautiful gym). The curriculum used for Project Active, titled *Active Living Every Day*, is available through Human Kinetics. This workbook contains information that your clients can use on their own or with your assistance. Topics such as setting goals, enlisting support, gaining confidence, and rewarding yourself are included.

After six months, both groups were much more active and still showed improvements in energy expenditure and cardiorespiratory fitness at two years (Dunn et al., 1999). Thus, regardless of the setting in which you work, we encourage you to think broadly about the type of activity to encourage. The lifestyle approach may work best for many people, especially in the earlier stages of motivational readiness for physical activity.

In addition to lifestyle approaches, it is important to consider incorporating muscle-strengthening activities. National guidelines now call for muscle-strengthening physical activities, focused on all major muscle groups, at least two days per week. This shift reflects the growing evidence of distinct benefits to muscle-strengthening activities for adults (e.g., 10-17% reduced risk of heart disease, cancer, diabetes, and all-cause mortality, independent of aerobic physical activity; Momma et al., 2022). When working with clients, you may wish to emphasize the additional advantages gained from combining aerobic and muscle-strengthening activities because meeting both aerobic and muscle-strengthening physical activity guidelines (vs. meeting just one or neither) has been associated with lower rates of coronary heart disease, diabetes, hypertension, and depression (Bennie, De Cocker, et al., 2019; Bennie, Teychenne, et al., 2019). Some subgroups of the population (e.g., individuals who are young, thin, affluent, male) are more likely to meet muscle-strengthening recommendations than others (Bennie et al., 2020), yet everyone can benefit from it and interest appears to be spreading. Latina participants in our past studies reported spontaneously increasing time spent in muscle-strengthening activities, even when enrolled in programs focused on aerobic physical activity (Benitez et al., 2022). Thus, your clients may be quite open to engaging in muscle-strengthening activities and benefit from a gentle nudge.

PROJECT STRIDE: A COMMUNITY-BASED STUDY

Given the epidemic of sedentary lifestyles, there is a need to develop effective, evidence-based interventions to promote physical activity that can be made widely available. Thus, we sought to test two delivery channels, telephone and print, to determine whether one was more effective than the other to promote physical activity among healthy, sedentary adults. Both intervention arms were guided by a motivationally tailored, theoretically driven computer expert system covering topics similar to those discussed in the previous studies.

Additionally, participants filled out questionnaires monthly during the first six months of the program and bimonthly during the second six months to provide the information needed to tailor their print or telephone feedback (Marcus, Napolitano, Lewis, et al., 2007). At six months, participants in both the telephone and print arms significantly increased their minutes of moderate-intensity physical activity compared to controls, with no differences between the intervention arms (mean minutes for print = 129.49 and for phone = 123.32). At 12 months, print participants reported a significantly greater number of moderate-intensity minutes than both telephone and control participants (mean minutes for print = 162.37 and for phone = 100.59; Marcus, Napolitano, King, et al., 2007). Results suggest that both telephone and print interventions enhance the adoption of physical activity among sedentary adults; however, print interventions may be particularly effective in maintaining physical activity in the longer term.

LEARNING HOW IT WORKS
Theory and Technology Enhancements

Participants greatly benefited from individualized physical activity feedback in the previously mentioned studies, yet most did not reach the national physical activity guidelines. Thus, subsequent studies explored providing additional support to help more individuals achieve health-enhancing levels of physical activity. How did we decide what to add?

Data on participant successes and preferences informed enhancements to the intervention (targeting additional social cognitive theory [SCT] constructs). Physical activity enjoyment, outcome expectations, and social support were not directly addressed in the *Seamos Saludables* program but improved more among participants with the highest increases in physical activity (Marcus et al., 2013, 2015; Pekmezi et al., 2012). In Seamos Activas II, the tailored reports were enhanced with feedback on participants' use of SCT constructs, including social support, enjoyment of activities done over the past month, and outcome expectations for physical activity, with strategies for decreasing negative and increasing positive expectations (Benitez et al., 2022). Tip sheets were provided, highlighting ways to increase enjoyment of physical activity, suggestions for fun physical activities to try, and different types of social support.

Another SCT strategy, self-regulation, was targeted through six months of daily text messages in response to participant requests for more accountability. The automated text messages encouraged physical activity tracking (2/wk) and goal setting (1/wk) and provided physical activity tips on other SCT constructs (4/wk). Table 5.1 shows a sample week of text messages. The goal-setting and self-monitoring texts were interactive. Participants answered questions about the minutes of physical activity per day they planned to do or had done that week and received automated feedback in response. For example:

Study: *"How many minutes of physical activity did you complete this week?"*
Participant: *"30"*
Study: *"Your physical activity goal this week was 30 minutes, and you reported doing 30 minutes. Great job reaching your goal this week!"*

Table 5.1 Sample Week of Text Messages Sent to Participants in the Enhanced Intervention Arm

Day	Theoretical construct targeted	Example of text message
Monday	Goal setting	Time to set your first exercise goal! What would you like your exercise goal to be this week? Thanks for setting a goal!
Tuesday	Social support	Ask [social supporter 2*] tonight to take a brisk walk with you in the morning—it will energize you for the day.
Wednesday	Environment	A quick Internet search can help you find fitness-related classes, events, and other information in your neighborhood.
Thursday	Self-monitoring	How many minutes of exercise have you done so far this week? Thanks for reporting your minutes of exercise!
Friday	Enjoyment	Choose active entertainment over passive entertainment.
Saturday	Social support	Make new friends! Exercise classes are great for meeting new people, which makes exercising more enjoyable.
Sunday	Self-monitoring & weekly goal feedback	How many total minutes of exercise did you do in the last 7 days? Thanks for reporting your minutes of exercise! Last week your goal was 150 min, and you reported 175 min of exercise.

*Participants were asked at baseline to name three potential sources of social support for physical activity.

The theory- and text-enhanced approaches to tailoring appear beneficial, especially when working with high-risk populations. Findings from Seamos Activas II indicated that the intervention enhancements helped more Latinas achieve national physical activity recommendations than the original intervention (57% vs. 44% at 6 months and 46.3% vs. 35.6% at 12 months, respectively). Small improvements in A1c (blood sugar levels), total cholesterol, and HDL and LDL cholesterol at six months were found among participants who received the enhanced intervention but not those who received the original intervention (Marcus et al., 2021).

STEP INTO MOTION: A COMMUNITY-BASED STUDY

Because >93 percent of Americans use the Internet (Pew Center), this represents an important channel for reaching the large population of sedentary people. Step Into Motion, a study based on the transtheoretical model, tested a web-based version of the protocol used in Project STRIDE (Marcus, Lewis, et al., 2007). The sample consisted of mostly underactive White (76.45%) women (84.2%). In this study 44.4 percent of the participants who received the tailored Internet-based intervention achieved the public health recommended levels of physical activity at six months (mean min/wk = 161.4), and 39.5 percent achieved these levels at 12 months (mean min/wk = 123.2). Numerous other studies have shown the Internet to be a viable tool that can be used to increase physical activity (Joseph et al., 2014; van den Berg et al., 2007) and help address related health disparities in underserved populations (Marcus et al., 2015, 2016). In the Pasos Hacia la Salud study, a Spanish-language, culturally adapted version of the individually tailored physical activity intervention website successfully increased physical activity in Latinas compared to a wellness contact control internet group (Marcus et al., 2016). Website engagement was strong in this sample (mean = 22 logins/12 months, SD = 28) and significantly associated with intervention success (Linke et al., 2019).

CONCLUSION

Overall, the studies described in this chapter suggest that using a stage-matched approach helps people progress toward more active lifestyles. These studies also demonstrate that matching interventions to participants' levels of motivational readiness is a more effective approach than using a one-treatment-fits-all approach, in which all people receive the same information regardless of their motivation to change their activity levels. Personalizing information to the individual was found to be important, and tailoring individualized physical activity feedback on additional SCT constructs (e.g., enjoyment, outcome expectations, social support) and incorporating technology (text messaging) produced greater improvements in physical activity outcomes. In the setting in which you work, accomplishing this personalization may be more or less feasible, but it is nonetheless important.

Another important finding of these studies is that effective programs need not be the traditional gym-based ones with which you may be quite familiar. Lifestyle activity programs, muscle-strengthening activities, and remote delivery channels are also quite effective in helping your clients achieve the improvements in health and physical activity they want. Moreover, in recent studies such programs have been successfully adapted to meet the unique intervention needs and preferences of diverse, underserved populations (Spanish-speaking Latino women and African American women in the Deep South).

Here ends part I, in which we focused on the theoretical backgrounds and tools for measuring motivational readiness for change. In part II we focus on applying the stages of motivational readiness for change model in individual, group, work, and community settings.

PART II

Applications

In part II we describe assessing patterns of physical activity and physical fitness, and we also examine applying the stages of motivational readiness for change model to various settings. We explain how to measure your clients' physical activity patterns and physical fitness as well as discuss how to apply the stages of the motivational readiness for change model to individual, group, worksite, and community settings. Then we discuss how you can apply these concepts to specific populations with whom you are working. Within this section we also provide exercises and worksheets that you can use in your physical activity programs and case studies that we hope will give you creative ideas of how you might use the information presented.

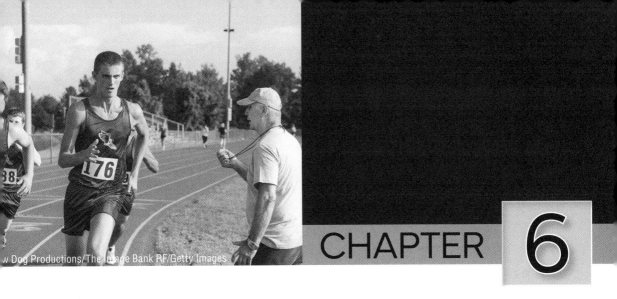

CHAPTER 6

Assessing Physical Activity Patterns and Physical Fitness

It is important for your clients to keep track of their participation in physical activity so that you know exactly what they are doing and can help them develop short- and long-term plans to reach their goals. Understanding patterns of behavior is an important first step in developing a plan to promote increases in physical activity behavior. Once you understand how clients spend their time, you can think of creative options to help them fit in some physical activity when they have been doing none and more activity when they have been doing a little.

In this chapter we describe a variety of ways to track activity patterns and help clients determine the intensity of their physical activity. We discuss the use of the stages of change questionnaire, introduced in chapter 2 (see questionnaire 2.1 in appendix A), to examine patterns of physical activity behavior. We introduce the idea of tracking physical activity habits with exercise logs and wearable devices (e.g., pedometers, wristbands). We describe using resting heart rate and time to walk half a mile (0.8 km) to measure physical fitness. We conclude by mentioning strategies for using these tools with more than one person at a time and refer to the following reports for more details on strategies for measuring physical activity (Dowd et al., 2018) and a review of the literature on the accuracy and acceptability of wrist-wearable activity trackers (Germini et al., 2022).

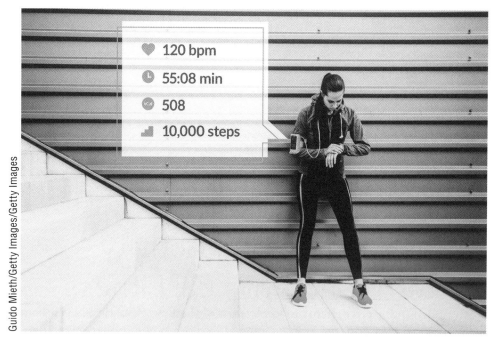

A smartwatch or wristband can both provide an assessment of your client's physical activity and serve as a source of client feedback toward reaching daily physical activity goals.

DISCOVERING PATTERNS OF PHYSICAL ACTIVITY BEHAVIOR

In chapter 2 we discussed determining a client's stage of motivational readiness for change. Although the stages of change questionnaire (questionnaire 2.1 in appendix A) does not allow you to learn about exact patterns of physical activity, such as the times of day people were active or whether they performed their activity all at once or in multiple short bouts throughout the day, it does allow you to assess their current activity level and intentions regarding future participation in physical activity. This questionnaire works well as a complement to other measures that provide detailed information about the number of minutes of physical activity per day and the types of activity performed. If global patterns of behavior and intention are most important in the setting in which you work, the stages of change questionnaire might be sufficient for your goals. This questionnaire is very brief, and studies have shown that scores on this measure correspond well with actual minutes of physical activity (Marcus & Simkin, 1993).

DETERMINING INTENSITY LEVEL

While light physical activity is better than sitting, your clients can receive more health benefits from gradually accelerating the pace and increasing both the frequency and intensity of moderate-vigorous physical activity. Therefore, one of your goals when working with clients is to help them understand the intensity with which they are performing physical activity to achieve health benefits. Some clients will be surprised to learn that they can gain many health benefits from moderate-intensity activities they already enjoy, such as raking leaves or dancing with their kids. Others might appreciate knowing that walking the dog a little faster provides extra mental and physical health perks. Table 6.1 shows categories of activities and examples of moderate-intensity and vigorous-intensity activities in each category. To help clients determine whether a given physical activity is of light, moderate, or vigorous intensity for them, you can use one of the methods discussed in the next three sections and/or a commercially available heart rate monitor.

Table 6.1 Examples of Activities of Varying Intensity Levels

Activity type	Moderate	Vigorous
Housework	Vacuuming carpet Cleaning windows Scrubbing floors	Moving furniture
Occupation	Walking briskly at work	Using heavy tools Loading and unloading a truck
Leisure	Line dancing	Salsa dancing
Gardening	Raking Mowing (push mower) Weeding	Shoveling Carrying moderate to heavy loads Tilling
Sports	Volleyball Table tennis Golf without a cart Tai chi Frisbee	Jumping rope Basketball Racquetball Soccer
Walking	Walking (3-4 mph [4-6 km/h])	Running Climbing stairs

Use the Talk Test

The talk test is one way to help your client understand what you mean by light-, moderate-, and vigorous-intensity activities. A person should be able to sing while doing light activities. When active at a moderate intensity, the person should be able to carry on a conversation comfortably. If a person is too winded or out of breath to carry on a conversation, the activity can be considered vigorous.

Monitor Target Heart Rate

Clients can also monitor their heart rate during physical activity to see whether they are within their desired intensity zone. For moderate-intensity physical activity, your clients should aim for a heart rate that is 60 to 76 percent of their maximum heart rate, which is based on their age. To estimate a person's maximum age-related heart rate, subtract their age from 220. Then calculate the 60 percent and 76 percent levels to obtain the moderate-intensity target range. For example, the estimated maximum age-related heart rate for a 50-year-old woman would be 220 − 50 years = 170 beats per minute (bpm). The target range for moderate-intensity activity would be as follows:

$$60\% \text{ level: } 170 \text{ bpm} \times 0.60 = 102 \text{ bpm}$$
$$76\% \text{ level: } 170 \text{ bpm} \times 0.76 = 129 \text{ bpm}$$

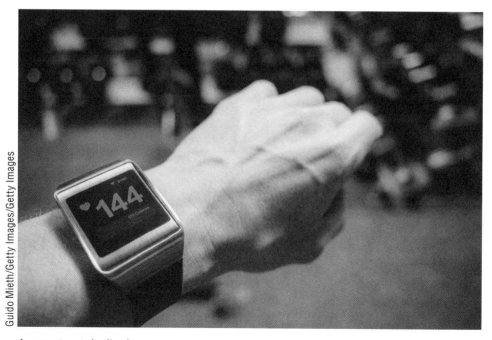

A smartwatch display.

You have determined that moderate-intensity physical activity for this 50-year-old woman requires a heart rate that remains between 102 and 129 bpm during physical activity. For vigorous activity, her heart rate should be 77 to 85 percent of her maximum age-related heart rate. We describe how to take heart rate by palpation later in this chapter in the Tracking the Resting Heart Rate section, but many find it simpler to use a commercially available heart rate monitor.

Commercially available heart rate monitors like the Apple Watch allow your clients to check their heart rate at any time with ease (e.g., using the Heart Rate app). The client just opens the app and waits for the Apple Watch to measure their heart rate (see picture of a smartwatch display). Resting, walking, breathing, workouts, and recovery rates are also available throughout the day. The Apple Watch has consistently shown good accuracy in measuring heart rate (Germini et al., 2022), even compared to other models (Fitbit Charge HR and Garmin Forerunner; Dooley et al., 2017), and among patients with cardiovascular disease (Falter et al., 2019).

Using Borg's Rating of Perceived Exertion

Perceived exertion is based on physical sensations your clients may experience during physical activity, including increased heart rate, increased breathing rate, sweating, and muscle fatigue. Although this is a subjective measure, it appears to be a good estimate of the actual heart rate (Borg, 1998). It also has an advantage over target heart rate because it does not require people to stop their activity to determine how hard they are working (Heyward, 2006). Using this scale, people can slow down or speed up their movement to adjust the intensity of their activity. The Borg scale also is the preferred method to determine intensity for people who are taking medications that affect heart rate or pulse (e.g., beta blockers, calcium channel blockers).

To determine physical activity intensity level, the person simply uses the Borg Rating of Perceived Exertion scale, which ranges from 6 (no exertion) to 20 (maximal exertion). Encourage clients to focus on their total level of exertion and not one specific aspect, such as leg pain or shortness of breath, and to base their rating on their own feeling of effort rather than on how it might compare to other people's. A rating of 9 (very light) is for low-intensity activities such as taking a slow walk at one's own pace. A rating of 12 to 14 (somewhat hard) suggests that the activity is being performed at moderate intensity, whereas a rating of 15 or higher (hard) is at vigorous intensity.

TRACKING TIME

Lack of time is a primary barrier for many people in their pursuit of a physically active lifestyle. To help your clients find more time to be physically active, you must find out how they spend their work and leisure time. This information can help you find times in the day when they are sedentary and could do some physical activity. Further, it can aid them in finding bouts of activity that can be lengthened. Only by understanding their activity patterns can you help them change these patterns. Have your clients choose two weekdays and one weekend day in an upcoming week during which to track their activities. Instruct them to use a smart phone application (or pen and paper) to record exactly what they do with their time on each of these three days.

In our past studies, participants have used mobile phone applications (e.g., Life in a Day) for measuring time use (see the following picture). This app was developed by the U.S. National Cancer Institute Division of Cancer Control and Population Sciences in collaboration with MEI Research, Ltd. and allows self-tracking of customizable activities (e.g., personal care, housecleaning, walking the dog). Participants reported finding the app easy to use (83%, 33/40) and preferable to logging activities via paper-and-pencil diaries (73%, 29/40). Similar time-use apps may help your clients become more aware of their habits and provide insights into how and when they could add physical activity to their daily lives (Ainsworth et al., 2018).

Once you understand how clients spend their time, you can work with them to turn time spent in sedentary behavior and light activity into time spent in moderate-intensity physical activity. For example, you can suggest that your clients replace time spent watching the kids play in the backyard with time spent bike riding or taking a nature walk with the kids. By reorganizing how they spend their time, they do not have to find more time for physical activity.

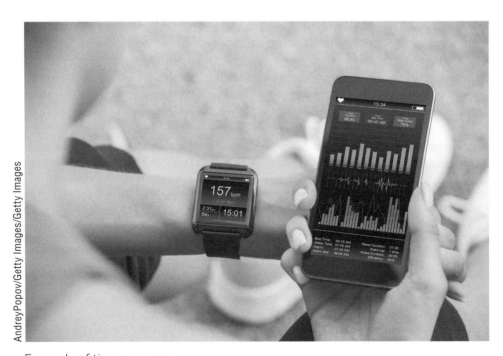

Example of time-use app.

Have your clients also keep track of how much time they spend in light-, moderate-, and vigorous-intensity activities. Wearable devices make this easy. Pedometers can be an excellent way to quantify amounts of activity. Although many come with extra features such as calculators of distance covered or calories burned, these are unnecessary and often inaccurate. The goal is for your clients to increase their activity. If they get too fixated on how far they have walked or how many calories they have burned, it may distract them from the goal and thus make meeting it less likely. Also, because distance and calorie calculations are often based on an average person, the values are often inaccurate for the person using them. For example, if your client is short and has a small stride, the readings may be off. Your client is best served with a simple version that just counts steps. We have used ACCUSPLIT pedometers in many of our studies, which cost from $20 to $50.

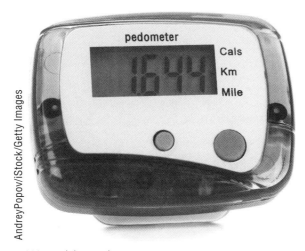

Wearable pedometer.

Pedometers look a lot like electronic pagers. They contain a small pendulum that moves each time the wearer takes a step. For the greatest accuracy, the wearer must keep the step counter centered over the left hipbone and lined up with the front crease of the slacks. The step counter *must* be firmly attached, so it is best worn on a belt or attached to the waistband of exercise shorts, pants, or undergarments. If your clients choose to wear the step counter on their underwear or tights, they should put it inside, not outside, the waistband. Also, they should be sure to remove the step counter before using the bathroom.

Advise your clients to put on the step counter first thing in the morning and keep it on until bedtime. When they take it off at bedtime, they should record the number of steps they took that day. Figure 6.1 provides a sample log sheet. They should be sure to reset the step counter back to zero for the next day of use.

Figure 6.1   Step counter log.

Week: _____

Day of week	Date	Step goal	Actual steps	Minutes of activity	Notes
Sunday					
Monday					
Tuesday					
Wednesday					
Thursday					
Friday					
Saturday					

From B. Marcus and D. Pekmezi, *Motivating People to be Physically Active*, 3rd ed. (Champaign, IL: Human Kinetics, 2025). Adapted by permission from S.N. Blair, A.L. Dunn, B.H. Marcus, et al., *Active Living Every Day*, 2nd ed. (Champaign, IL: Human Kinetics, 2011).

After your clients have recorded their steps for a week, they can calculate their average steps per day. Then you can help them set a reasonable goal and devise a plan to increase their steps to reach that goal. Adults in America, Canada, and other Western nations average about 5117 steps per day (Bassett et al., 2010). The long-term goal we usually recommend is 10,000 steps per day, but this information came from a 1960s Japanese pedometer marketing campaign, not science. Lower amounts have produced health benefits. For example, recent studies have shown that people who took 7,000 steps per day had a 50 percent to 70 percent lower risk of premature death compared to those who took less than 7,000 steps per day (Paluch et al., 2021). Similar advantages (40% reduced risk of premature death) were found for 4,400 versus 2,700 (or less) steps per day (Lee et al., 2019). Thus, if your client is getting about 5,000 steps a day, adding an extra 2,000 to 3,000 steps could improve longevity.

Moreover, for a client who is taking only 2,500 steps per day, you may *not* want to talk about a long-term goal of obtaining 10,000 steps per day. Rather, you may want to set a goal of 5,000 steps per day, which is more easily attainable for a person at that activity level. Once the client has met this goal, the two of you can reevaluate and set the next goal. You may want to create a form to track their progress over time, such as the example in figure 6.2. A simple graph that you or your client fills out can be a useful way to demonstrate that there has been great progress or that there is some room for improvement.

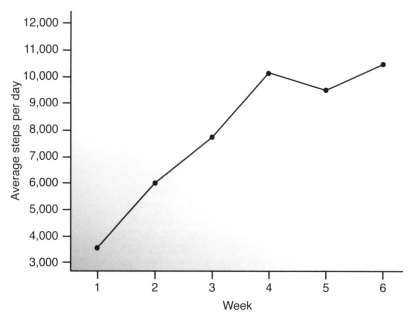

Figure 6.2 A weekly goal chart showing the average number of steps taken per day can motivate your clients to increase the number of steps they take per day.

Accelerometers

Accelerometers capture body movement from several different axes and can measure the acceleration of the device from side to side (lateral), up and down (longitudinal), and front to back (vertical).

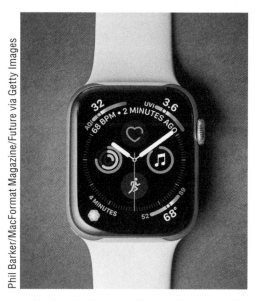

An accelerometer can display daily steps, floors climbed, miles, calories expended, and active minutes.

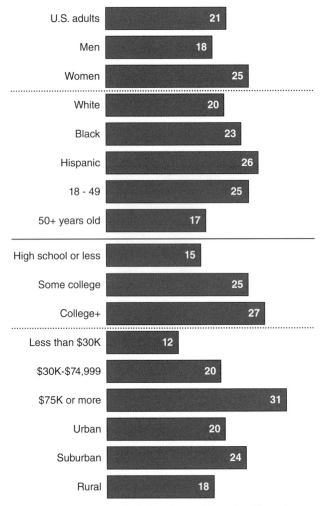

Figure 6.3 Survey conducted by Pew Research Center about adults wearing fitness trackers.

From Pew Research Center. Available: https://www.pewresearch.org/short-reads/2020/01/09/about-one-in-five-americans-use-a-smart-watch-or-fitness-tracker

Most smart phones come with accelerometers and can be used to track steps if the client remembers to keep the phone on their person. Many commercially available wristbands are also available that track steps using accelerometers. Wristbands are easy to see and make great visual prompts to be active. Clients can upload the data and view graphical displays of their progress over time using smart phone apps.

Wearables are rising in popularity, with almost 21 percent of American adults reporting regularly wearing a smart watch or wearable fitness tracker, according to the Pew Research Center (figure 6.3). Survey data from 4,272 U.S. adults in 2020 also indicated that device use varies among subgroups. Individuals with household incomes less than $75,000 and college degrees are adopting this technology at higher rates than those with lower household incomes and education levels. Individuals diagnosed and/or at risk for cardiovascular disease have also reported lower rates of using wearable devices (18% and 26%, respectively; vs. 29% for general U.S. population; Dhingra et al., 2023). Thus, you should consider discussing wearables with clients, as those who could benefit most from such devices might be missing out.

Light activity may be important too. This data can give you some ideas on how to break up sitting time and turn some of this light activity into moderate-intensity activity. For example, you can set "sitting alerts" with commercially available smart phone apps or even use an alarm on your phone (or use a smart phone app) to remind you to stand up and move if you have been sitting too long. Strolling around the park could be increased to brisk walking. If your clients are not sure whether the activity was light, moderate, or vigorous, they should consider whether the effort was more like a slow walk at two miles (3.2 km) per hour (light activity), a brisk walk at three to four miles (4.8 to 6.4 km) per hour (moderate activity), or a run (vigorous activity). At the end of each week, you or your clients can examine time spent in each

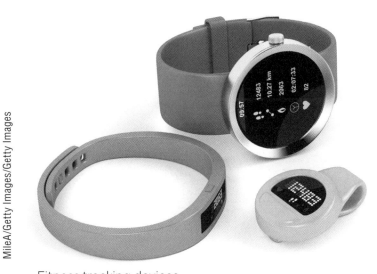

Fitness tracking devices.

activity category and use this information to set realistic goals for improving their level of physical activity, to design a specific activity program, and to determine whether they have met their goals.

Old-school methods still work!

If your clients do not embrace wearables, they can always just record their minutes of moderate- and vigorous-intensity physical activity using a pen and paper log (figure 6.4). If your clients are using this "old-school" approach, encourage them to log daily rather than wait and try to recall a week's worth of physical activity at once.

After your clients track their physical activity habits, it is time to put this information to work to help them become more active. First, look for patterns in the tracking forms that your clients have filled out. Do your clients tend to be sedentary for the entire workday? If so, a 10-minute walk once each workday might be a great way to help them on their way to a more active lifestyle. Another pattern to look for is time spent in light activity. Help your clients turn strolls into brisk walks, elevator rides into stair climbing, and light yard work into more vigorous yard work. Tracking activity will help you and your clients set goals for becoming more active over time and reaching the national physical activity guidelines.

Figure 6.4   Blank activity tracking sheet.

MVPA min/day _____

Steps _____

FEBRUARY, 2024

Sun.	Mon.	Tues.	Wed.	Thurs.	Fri.	Sat.
				01	02	03
				Minutes of moderate-vigorous physical activity ____	Minutes of moderate-vigorous physical activity ____	Minutes of moderate-vigorous physical activity ____
04	05	06	07	08	09	10
Minutes of moderate-vigorous physical activity ____	Minutes of moderate-vigorous physical activity ____	Minutes of moderate-vigorous physical activity ____	Minutes of moderate-vigorous physical activity ____	Minutes of moderate-vigorous physical activity ____	Minutes of moderate-vigorous physical activity ____	Minutes of moderate-vigorous physical activity ____

From B. Marcus and D. Pekmezi, *Motivating People to be Physically Active,* 3rd ed. (Champaign, IL: Human Kinetics, 2025).

LEARNING HOW IT WORKS
Which Activity Tracker Should I Recommend to My Client?

There are many considerations when picking the right activity tracker for your client. First is accuracy. Pedometers tend to underestimate steps compared to direct observation and accelerometers. Most pedometers simply track the up-and-down movement of the hips that occurs each time you take a step. Accelerometers are more sensitive and can detect movement from side to side (lateral), up and down (longitudinal), and front to back (vertical). Activity monitors (Fitbit Charge and Fitbit Charge HR) have consistently shown good accuracy for step counts (Germini et al., 2022) but tend to slightly overestimate distance traveled and underestimate time spent by activity type compared to direct observation (Dowd et al., 2018). If you have concerns about the accuracy of a device, walk 20 steps with it on and then check the reading. If the reading is not accurate, consider adjustments to the positioning of the pedometer or accelerometer.

Here are some questions to ask when deciding which device to recommend to your client:

- Does your client like fancy technology? Or does your client prefer to keep things simple?
- Does your client have a smart phone? Will or can your client download apps?
- Is cost an issue?
- Does your client prefer wearing devices on the hip or wrist?

Female participants in our past studies have reported preferring wristbands, describing them as more fashionable and flattering than hip-worn devices. On the other hand, several older participants in the DIAL study had difficulties setting up their fitness tracker monitors and requested simpler pedometers (Brown et al., 2021). Moreover, individuals who are not accustomed to wearing a watch or have sensitive skin (or even develop minor skin rashes) may take time to acclimate to wristbands. Finally, price can be an important practical consideration. Pedometers are generally more reasonably priced than activity monitors. In sum, when deciding which activity tracking strategy to recommend to your clients, consider which device they can and will actually use!

Here is an example of how to use activity tracking with a sedentary client. Natalie is a 43-year-old mother of two who works as a schoolteacher. She is interested in increasing her physical activity level to maintain her weight and improve her energy level so she can keep up with her kids. Her fitness tracker weekly progress report, presented in figure 6.5, shows very little activity (few steps/day) during the weekdays. Natalie describes being very busy with work during the week and spending most school days sitting or doing light-intensity activity. Thus, one important strategy for working with Natalie is to acknowledge limited time on weekdays and determine how to break up sitting and performing light activities at a brisker, more moder-

(continued)

> **Which Activity Tracker Should I Recommend to My Client?** *(continued)*
>
> ate intensity. For example, Natalie could park at the back of the lot when she arrives at work in the morning to get more steps (or even ride her bike to school). Once at work, she could take activity breaks between lessons (stretch, march in place) in the classroom and walk around the playground while supervising recess (instead of sitting). In the evenings, she could make family time more active by playing tag or active video games with her kids. Activity tracking helped her see that rather than squeezing in more activity, she could break up sitting time, accumulate more steps, and exchange light-intensity activities for moderate-intensity ones.

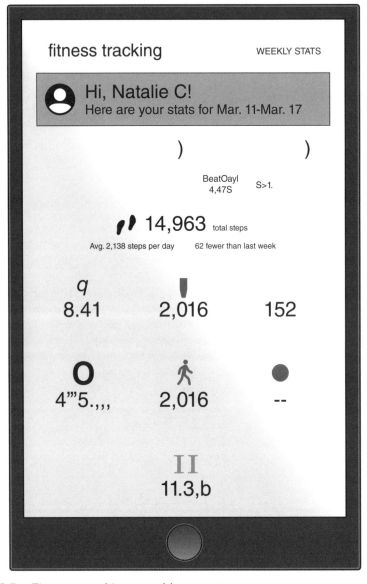

Figure 6.5 Fitness tracking weekly report.

ASSESSING FITNESS

We have described means for measuring your clients' time spent engaging in physical activities and patterns of behavior. Understanding these patterns is critical to helping them see more benefits and fewer barriers to living an active lifestyle and to enhancing their motivation to become more physically active. However, actual physical fitness is also an important factor in increasing clients' levels of physical activity.

If a client has a very high resting heart rate and cannot walk even half a mile (0.8 km) without becoming breathless, the client will need to start an activity program very slowly, even if there is considerable motivation to change. For example, this client could begin performing 2-minute bouts of activity and then slowly increase to 5- and then 10-minute bouts. On the other hand, if your client is fit enough to easily accomplish a half-mile (0.8 km) walk but lack of time is a barrier, your physical activity plan may focus more on rearranging the schedule. You can encourage this client to turn light activity into moderate-intensity activity and to string short bouts of activity together into longer bouts of activity without necessarily adding to the busy day. Activity pattern assessment and physical fitness assessment work together to help you customize a program that will best meet your client's needs.

It is important to develop a plan that your client can start and maintain, thereby enhancing the likelihood that your client will eventually be active daily. We will now give you some simple strategies for assessing your client's fitness level. The following two sections give detailed information about assessing a client's physical fitness, physical readiness for more activity, or both (refer to Heyward, 2006, for more in-depth information on physical fitness assessment).

Tracking the Resting Heart Rate

One of the simplest ways to gauge changes in fitness is to track the resting heart rate (bpm). As clients' fitness improves, their resting heart rate slows down. When people increase their fitness level, their hearts get stronger and can pump more blood with each beat compared to when they are less fit.

Your clients may not know how to measure their resting heart rate. The easiest place to find a pulse is on the inside of the wrist, just below the thumb. Help your clients learn how to place their index and middle fingers lightly against the artery at that location. They may need to move their fingers around a bit until they can feel the rhythmic beat of their pulse. Next, using a second hand on a watch or a stopwatch, have them count how many times their heart beats in one minute. Then they can record it on a form like the one shown in figure 6.6. Ideally, to ensure the accuracy of this measure, advise your clients to record their heart rate first thing in the morning, before getting out of bed, or before they have had any coffee or cigarettes, as either of these stimulants could greatly affect their resting heart rate. As previously mentioned, smart phone applications and fitness bands can also be used to monitor heart rate.

Figure 6.6   Resting heart rate log.

Date	Resting heart rate	Notes

From B. Marcus and D. Pekmezi, *Motivating People to be Physically Active,* 3rd ed. (Champaign, IL: Human Kinetics, 2025).

Depending on your situation and your plans for working with your clients, you may prefer to measure and record the clients' resting heart rate rather than have them do it. If your client has numerous risk factors for heart disease and has repeatedly tried but failed to become more active, you may want to be more proactive. However, if you are working with a more motivated person who wants to work with you only briefly and then work more independently, it is probably best to give the client more autonomy from the beginning and teach the client how to record the heart rate.

Every month (or whatever interval makes sense in your situation), have your clients measure and record their resting heart rate. If they are participating in physical activity regularly, their resting heart rate should decrease over time. Depending on the circumstances, you may also want your clients to record whether they are experiencing any extreme emotions, such as stress, worry, or sadness. Strong emotional responses can affect heart rate and may help you interpret unexpected patterns in heart rate over time.

Walking Test

A simple and inexpensive way to assess changes in fitness is a walking test. Your clients will need access to a half-mile (0.8 km) track, or they can map their own half-mile (0.8 km) route. Be sure they warm up first by walking slowly for a few minutes. Then you can time them or have them time themselves as they walk this route as quickly as possible. In some settings, it may be efficient for a group of people (e.g., employees) to perform this test at the same time. You or your clients should record how long it takes to walk the half mile (0.8 km) and their heart rate immediately after they finish. This will help you determine how hard they were working while they walked that distance (figure 6.7). Advise your clients to refrain from cigarette smoking and coffee and soft drink consumption for at least one hour prior to this walking test because these stimulants can raise the heart rate. Clients should repeat this test in approximately three months to determine their progress.

Chapter 6   Assessing Physical Activity Patterns and Physical Fitness   **85**

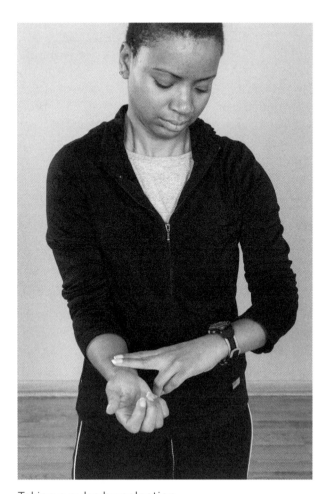

Taking a pulse by palpation.

Figure 6.7   Walking test log.

Date	Time to walk half mile (minutes and seconds)	Heart rate at end

From B. Marcus and D. Pekmezi, *Motivating People to be Physically Active,* 3rd ed. (Champaign, IL: Human Kinetics, 2025). Reprinted by permission from S.N. Blair et al., *Active Living Every Day* (Champaign, IL: Human Kinetics, 2001).

Two-Minute Step Test

Perhaps you and your client do not have access to a half-mile (0.8 km) track. You may be short on time or facing inclement weather. In this case, you should consider a brief physical function test that can be conducted indoors, such as the two-minute step test (Rikli et al., 1999). This protocol (detailed in Learning How It Works) is particularly appropriate when working with clients who are older, inactive, and living with medical conditions (i.e., not up for a half-mile [0.8 km] walk). While the two-minute step test is typically done in person, we recently adapted this instrument for virtual use and demonstrated the validity and reliability of the remote protocol (Hoenemeyer et al., 2022).

LEARNING HOW IT WORKS
Measuring Physical Function in Tight Spaces? Try the Two-Minute Step Test

Instructions: For this test, the administrator will need a tape measure, masking or painters' tape, a stopwatch, and a clicker.

Establish the knee lift height:

1. Have the participant stand against the wall. Measure from the top of the hip bone (iliac crest) to the kneecap (patella). Find the halfway point between the two.
2. Measure from this halfway point to the ground with the tape measure.
3. Place a mark on the wall with masking tape at the height from the ground to the participant's mid-thigh. The participant is aiming to lift their knees to this marker.

Instructions to the participant from the person administering the test:

1. When I say, "Go [or start], step up and down, lifting your knees to this mark on the wall." *Point to the marker on the wall and demonstrate stepping up and down.*
2. "Continue to step as fast as you can for two minutes."
3. "If you get tired, please slow down or stop and rest. You can take as many breaks as you need."
4. "I will let you know when you have reached two minutes."

Instructions for the person administering the test:

1. Start the stopwatch once you have instructed the participant to begin.
2. Using the clicker, count the total number of times the RIGHT knee reaches the tape level in two minutes.

3. Stop the stopwatch at two minutes.
4. Record the total number of times the right knee meets the tape on your assessment sheet.

Distance from hip bone to kneecap: _____ cm

Midway distance between hip bone and kneecap to floor: _____ cm

Total number of steps (Number of times *right* knee rises to mark): _____

Virtual administration via video-conferencing call (requires a partner): A partner is asked to locate the iliac crest (hip bone), then use the vinyl tape measure to record the distance to the top of the patella (knee) and call it out to the assessor. The assessor calculates the midpoint, which is denoted by a sticker. The partner is then asked to measure the distance from the sticker to the floor and call out the value to the assessor. The assessor records this value for future testing and then instructs the partner to measure this distance to the floor against a wall and to mark it with another sticker. Upon the command to start, the participant marches in place for two minutes, making sure to bring their knees up to the sticker. The participant is instructed not to talk and to take breaks and brace against the wall if needed while the timer continues (the partner also is instructed to "spot" the participant as needed). The number of steps reaching the mark is counted.

CONCLUSION

In this chapter we explained why it is important to understand and track your clients' physical activity patterns and physical fitness and function, and we provided you with strategies that will be helpful in accomplishing these objectives. We discussed various tools (pedometers, wristbands, smart phone applications, etc.) for tracking your clients' activity habits because tracking these variables is critical in helping them create realistic, measurable goals for becoming more active. Trends, advantages, and disadvantages of various activity trackers are presented, along with practical considerations for selecting the methods that will work best for your client. Common techniques for monitoring heart rate, time use, and sedentary behaviors were explored, which can help clients gauge and increase the intensity of daily activities (e.g., walk more briskly), break up sitting time, and find opportunities for integrating more physical activity bouts into their schedule. Such habits will result in improvements in physical fitness and function for your clients, which can be assessed through the protocols outlined in the chapter (half-mile [0.8 km] walk, 2-minute step test). We also described how to use the methods presented in this chapter with more than one client at a time. Now that you are familiar with assessment methods, you are ready to learn about applying the stages of change model in your work with clients.

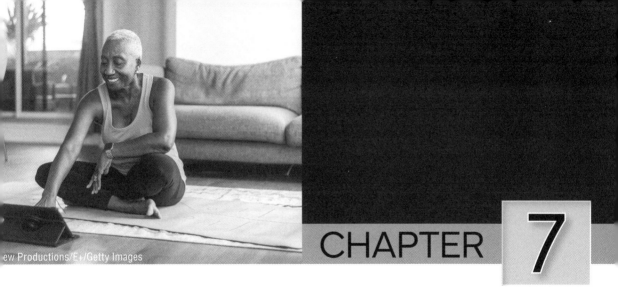

CHAPTER 7

Using the Stages Model in Individual Counseling

The Transtheoretical model was originally developed by observing how people change behavior on their own. The goal was to discover the key ingredients in behavior change so that counselors and therapists could use these strategies to help people change their behaviors. This chapter on applying the stages of change model focuses on individual counseling. Professionals can help clients set goals for activity, address problems that arise, and use clients' past histories of behavior change to achieve their current goals.

In this chapter we describe how to assess clients' physical and psychological readiness to engage in physical activity. We explain why it is important to examine clients' experiences with changing habits and how to help them solve problems that may be getting in the way of becoming more active. We also describe strategies for enhancing clients' confidence that they can change their behavior and for helping them set realistic goals for behavior change. Each of these issues is pertinent at all stages of motivational readiness because of the cyclical nature of behavior change. Therefore, many of the areas described in this chapter need to be addressed repeatedly during the initiation, adoption, and maintenance of physical activity habits. However, these topics are addressed slightly differently for people at each stage. The Stage-Specific Strategies section at the end of this chapter provides some ideas for how you can apply each topic at each stage of motivational readiness when working with individuals. One of the first steps in individual counseling is to assess the client's stage of motivational readiness for physical activity. You should keep this stage in mind as you work with the client using the strategies discussed in this chapter.

PHYSICAL READINESS

In chapter 1 we described the numerous health benefits of an active lifestyle. Although most people benefit from participating in programs of regular physical activity, those with health problems may need more medical supervision than you or your facility can provide. Thus, it is important to first assess your client's physical readiness for physical activity before embarking on specific physical activity counseling. Recommendations on screening participants for readiness for exercise participation have shifted from emphasizing age cutoffs, risk factor profiling, and risk stratification terminology (i.e., low, moderate, high) to focusing on the individual's current activity level; known cardiovascular (CVD), metabolic, or renal disease; potential signs or symptoms of CVD; and the anticipated exercise intensity (all factors associated with risk for exercise-related acute cardiovascular events; Franklin et al., 2020).

RISK MODULATOR CATEGORY
Potential Risk Modulators of Exercise-Related Acute Cardiovascular Events

Individual's current level of activity

Presence of signs and symptoms suggestive of CVD

Pain or discomfort at rest or with physical exertion in the chest, neck, jaw, arms, or other areas that could result from myocardial ischemia
- Unusual shortness of breath
- Lightheadedness
- Ankle swelling
- Awareness of a rapid or irregular heartbeat
- Burning or cramping sensations in the lower extremities when walking short distances

Known CVD, metabolic, or renal disease
- Diabetes (type 1 and type 2 diabetes mellitus)
- angina pectoris, previous myocardial infarction, coronary revascularization, heart surgery, pacemaker, valve disease, heart failure, structural heart disease

Desired exercise intensity

Adapted by permission from M. Armstrong et al., "Preparticipation Screen before Physical Activity in Community Lifestyle Interventions," *Translational Journal of the ACSM* 3, no. 22 (2018): 176-180.

Depending on your professional training, you may or may not feel comfortable addressing safety with your client. In general, exercising at a moderate intensity (as opposed to vigorously) is safe. A medical exam or stress test is not required before increasing moderate-intensity physical activities for most people. However, going straight "from couch to 5K" with vigorous-intensity physical activity is not advisable, because this can increase the risk of sudden cardiac death and acute myocardial infarction in predisposed individuals (Franklin et al., 2020). In fact, people with conditions such as heart disease should check with their doctors before beginning to exercise even at a moderate intensity. One often-used method of determining whether a person can safely increase activity is the Physical Activity Readiness Questionnaire (PAR-Q; figure 7.1). Your client should read the questionnaire carefully and answer each yes-or-no question honestly.

2023 PAR-Q+

The Physical Activity Readiness Questionnaire for Everyone

The health benefits of regular physical activity are clear; more people should engage in physical activity every day of the week. Participating in physical activity is very safe for MOST people. This questionnaire will tell you whether it is necessary for you to seek further advice from your doctor OR a qualified exercise professional before becoming more physically active.

GENERAL HEALTH QUESTIONS

Please read the 7 questions below carefully and answer each one honestly: check YES or NO.	YES	NO
1) Has your doctor ever said that you have a heart condition ☐ OR high blood pressure ☐?	☐	☐
2) Do you feel pain in your chest at rest, during your daily activities of living, OR when you do physical activity?	☐	☐
3) Do you lose balance because of dizziness OR have you lost consciousness in the last 12 months? Please answer NO if your dizziness was associated with over-breathing (including during vigorous exercise).	☐	☐
4) Have you ever been diagnosed with another chronic medical condition (other than heart disease or high blood pressure)? PLEASE LIST CONDITION(S) HERE: _____	☐	☐
5) Are you currently taking prescribed medications for a chronic medical condition? PLEASE LIST CONDITION(S) AND MEDICATIONS HERE: _____	☐	☐
6) Do you currently have (or have had within the past 12 months) a bone, joint, or soft tissue (muscle, ligament, or tendon) problem that could be made worse by becoming more physically active? Please answer NO if you had a problem in the past, but it does not limit your current ability to be physically active. PLEASE LIST CONDITION(S) HERE: _____	☐	☐
7) Has your doctor ever said that you should only do medically supervised physical activity?	☐	☐

If you answered NO to all of the questions above, you are cleared for physical activity.
Please sign the PARTICIPANT DECLARATION. You do not need to complete Pages 2 and 3.

- Start becoming much more physically active – start slowly and build up gradually.
- Follow Global Physical Activity Guidelines for your age (https://www.who.int/publications/i/item/9789240015128).
- You may take part in a health and fitness appraisal.
- If you are over the age of 45 yr and NOT accustomed to regular vigorous to maximal effort exercise, consult a qualified exercise professional before engaging in this intensity of exercise.
- If you have any further questions, contact a qualified exercise professional.

PARTICIPANT DECLARATION

If you are less than the legal age required for consent or require the assent of a care provider, your parent, guardian or care provider must also sign this form.

I, the undersigned, have read, understood to my full satisfaction and completed this questionnaire. I acknowledge that this physical activity clearance is valid for a maximum of 12 months from the date it is completed and becomes invalid if my condition changes. I also acknowledge that the community/fitness center may retain a copy of this form for its records. In these instances, it will maintain the confidentiality of the same, complying with applicable law.

NAME _____ DATE _____

SIGNATURE _____ WITNESS _____

SIGNATURE OF PARENT/GUARDIAN/CARE PROVIDER _____

If you answered YES to one or more of the questions above, COMPLETE PAGES 2 AND 3.

⚠ **Delay becoming more active if:**
- You have a temporary illness such as a cold or fever; it is best to wait until you feel better.
- You are pregnant - talk to your health care practitioner, your physician, a qualified exercise professional, and/or complete the ePARmed-X+ at www.eparmedx.com before becoming more physically active.
- Your health changes - answer the questions on Pages 2 and 3 of this document and/or talk to your doctor or a qualified exercise professional before continuing with any physical activity program.

Copyright © 2023 PAR-Q+ Collaboration 1 / 4
01-11-2022

Figure 7.1 Page one of the Physical Activity Readiness Questionnaire.

Reprinted with permission from the PAR-Q+ Collaboration and the authors of the PAR-Q+ (Dr. Darren Warburton, Dr. Norman Gledhill, Dr. Veronica Jamnik, and Dr. Shannon Bredin).

Clients who answer yes to one or more questions on the PAR-Q should speak with their doctors before increasing their physical activity. They should be sure to tell their doctors the specific questions to which they answered yes.

Clients who answer no to all the questions can begin activity slowly and increase it gradually, but may require guidance on how to do this. If you work with clients for more than six months, periodically re-administer the PAR-Q. If clients answer yes to any of the questions, have them contact their doctors.

People who come to you for help are likely to be sedentary; therefore, they should begin with moderate (not vigorous) intensity activities. Gradually progressing the intensity of exercise regimens allows newcomers to build up cardiorespiratory respiratory fitness and reduce their risks for exercise-related acute cardiac events (Franklin et al., 2020).

PHYSICAL ACTIVITY HISTORY

Once you have determined that clients can safely increase their physical activity, it is helpful to learn more about their experiences with physical activity. Questionnaire 7.1 in appendix A will help you determine how long it has been since they were more physically active, some reasons they stopped being physically active in the past, and the activities they may have previously enjoyed. The information from this questionnaire can be useful as you plan individual or group programs. For clients who are currently inactive or underactive, we encourage you to look for patterns in their responses to this questionnaire so that you can prevent similar relapses from occurring this time. You also may want to re-administer this questionnaire as necessary to be aware of clients' shifting priorities.

PSYCHOLOGICAL READINESS

Psychological readiness, not physical readiness, is likely to be the main barrier to activity for most of your clients. Although you might not see a lot of stage 1 people in the setting in which you work, chances are good that you see many stage 2 clients—people who keep meaning to start some physical activity but never get around to it. You may also see people in stage 3 who do some physical activity but have not quite figured out how to make it a habit. They may need your help increasing the frequency and duration of their physical activity to obtain important health benefits. Your task with all your clients is to aid them in moving through the stages of change and help them avoid pitfalls on what can be an arduous journey. You must help them understand how their behavior regarding physical activity is like other behaviors they have succeeded in changing in the past. You can help them examine the benefits of and barriers to changing their behavior and assist them in solving problems that arise when they try to change their physical activity habits. You also can aid them in building confidence in themselves and in setting realistic goals that they can achieve to make them feel proud and successful.

Personal Successes and Past Behavior Change

Some clients may want to be more active but tell you that they do not believe they can succeed. The idea of changing their whole lives to become more active is overwhelming. One very effective tool for working with clients like these is to sidestep the issue of physical activity initially. Instead, start off by helping them recall some other lifestyle change they made, with or without professional help. This is key because past behavior is the single strongest predictor of future behavior. Helping clients recall past successes is likely to empower them to make positive changes in their physical activity habits.

Have your clients take a few minutes to relate one or more success stories—a healthy habit they have adopted or an unhealthy habit they have stopped. Then ask them to think about why they could make the change. What helped them succeed? What got in their way? For example, if a client quit smoking by setting their 40th birthday as the quit date and receiving support from family, friends, and coworkers, this gives you both a lot of information that might help the client start a program of regular physical activity. Figure 7.2 is an example of a form you and your client might use to record these successes.

Figure 7.2 Record of past successes.

Habits I've changed
1.
2.
3.
Things that helped me succeed
1.
2.
3.
Obstacles that got in my way
1.
2.
3.

From B. Marcus and D. Pekmezi, *Motivating People to be Physically Active*, 3rd ed. (Champaign, IL: Human Kinetics, 2025).

Once you and your client have discussed past successes and how they were achieved, you should have a lot of useful information about the strategies that work and do not work for your client. This information can help you work with your client's areas of strength (e.g., a lot of supportive friends) and deal with challenges (e.g., long work hours). In this way you can create a program that is uniquely suited to your client and, thus, extremely likely to help with goal achievement.

> ### *LEARNING HOW IT WORKS*
> **Learning From Past Efforts at Behavior Change**
>
> Sometimes there is a lot that can be learned from past efforts at behavior change. For example, your client is completely sedentary and has no history of being physically active. However, the client demonstrated success in behavior changes in other areas before (reducing caffeine intake). This is useful information. Investigate further!
>
> First, what were your client's previous motivations for behavior change?
>
> Perhaps the motivation to change a behavior (cut back on caffeine) was to help improve health and quality of life (fewer headaches). If so, you may want to emphasize how increasing physical activity may also improve health and quality of life. You can use information on the client's priorities to help align the new health behavior with what is personally important.
>
> Who convinced the client to consider behavior change?
>
> If you learn that the client's past success with behavior change began with the primary care physician saying that decreased caffeine consumption might help decrease the frequency and intensity of headaches, this may give you insights into who the client listens to and how to best proceed. The client may benefit from speaking to this physician about the benefits of a more active lifestyle.
>
> What behavior change strategies were more or less helpful last time?
>
> Perhaps your client radically decreased the amount of caffeine consumed by gradually switching to decaffeinated coffee at work. Healthy substitutions worked before; maybe they could work again. If the client is mostly sedentary at the office, perhaps trying to take a few extra steps during work breaks (rather than checking social media) could be a starting point.
>
> Who was supportive of behavior change last time? Who was not?
>
> The client was able to maintain a caffeine-free lifestyle with phone calls, texts, and emails from friends over the next two weeks. Interestingly, the spouse continued to offer regular coffee and suggested that decaf was not "real" coffee. This information about your client's past provides many important clues for helping change physical activity behavior. The spouse may or may not support the client's desire to be more active. However, support from friends appears to have worked before. Where are those friends now? How can they be mobilized to walk with your client and encourage more activity?

Readiness to Change Physical Activity Habits

Some people believe that we just need to make up our minds to do something, and then we can do it, relying on a lot of willpower in the process. However, most behavior change happens slowly, and lasting behavior change occurs only when a person is motivated to change. Some people can make major lifestyle changes on their own, whereas many others need help, often from professionals like you.

How do clients know that they are ready to change a behavior? One way is to ask themselves, "What will I get as a result of making this behavior change?" or "What are the benefits of change?" If they cannot come up with at least a few key benefits, they are unlikely to accomplish even short-term change at this point. Have them take a few moments to write down their reasons for wanting to change their activity habits. This exercise is useful for clients at all stages of motivational readiness (even people in stage 1 can list many reasons to become more active; they just have not acted on them) because understanding the benefits of exercise is critical for adopting and maintaining a physically active lifestyle.

Another important component of changing behavior is determining what your client will have to give up or what they will find unpleasant if they make a change. It is unrealistic to think that a person can make a major life transition (e.g., go from inactive to regularly active) without having some aspects of the process be annoying or frustrating. Barriers to behavior change might impede your client's best-laid plans. For example, if your client is worried that the family will feel burdened or neglected because of spending time on physical activity, you should discuss this. Have the client take a few minutes to make a list of any barriers to physical activity behavior change. Figures 7.3 and 7.4 present sample forms for listing both the benefits of and barriers to physical activity.

With your client, look over the list of barriers to physical activity and examine the number and nature of the barriers. Discuss the degree to which each factor affects participation in physical activity (e.g., very much, somewhat, not at all) to determine which is the most important (and if any can be omitted from the list). This will help you gauge where to address barriers. The next section describes one strategy for problem-solving.

Figure 7.3 Record of benefits of physical activity.

Benefits of physical activity
1.
2.
3.
4.
5.
6.
7.
8.

From B. Marcus and D. Pekmezi, *Motivating People to be Physically Active,* 3rd ed. (Champaign, IL: Human Kinetics, 2025).

Figure 7.4 Record of barriers to physical activity.

Barriers to physical activity
1.
2.
3.
4.
5.
6.
7.
8.

From B. Marcus and D. Pekmezi, *Motivating People to be Physically Active*, 3rd ed. (Champaign, IL: Human Kinetics, 2025).

The IDEA Approach to Problem-Solving

Once your clients have identified their barriers to being physically active, the next step is to help them use some simple problem-solving skills. Problem-solving means thinking creatively about the most effective solution to use when a problem gets in the way. Flexible thinking is key. Encourage your clients to think outside the box when coming up with solutions. Sometimes the most absurd solution actually works best! Once they have come up with a variety of possible solutions, help them choose one to try out first; you can determine later how well it worked. They should pick a good time to implement their solutions to enhance the likelihood of success. Emphasize that finding out that one solution does not work is not bad news. This information can help you both find a better solution that not only works but also can be maintained over time. The concept of looking for alternative solutions when one does not pan out helps to counter all-or-nothing thinking, which often keeps a person from making change (e.g., "I can't find an hour per day to walk right now, so I'll wait until work slows down this summer").

The IDEA technique is a simple problem-solving approach that has worked well in a number of our studies and with many clients. The acronym stands for *identify* the problem, *develop* a list of solutions, *evaluate* the solutions, and *analyze* how well the plan worked. It is easy to implement and can be helpful to all clients, especially those who are struggling to see past their barriers to behavior change. The goal is to help clients discover new options and feel less "stuck" in making desired changes to their current situations.

Identify the Problem

The first step of the IDEA approach is to have your client select one barrier and write it down on the IDEA form in figure 7.5 found at the end of this chapter. Ask your clients to think about how this barrier specifically keeps them from being active. Next, ask them to write down the most important details about this personal barrier. For example, their stated barrier may be "not having a gym membership," but their primary concern is personal safety when exercising in their neighborhood.

Figure 7.5 IDEA form

Identify a barrier that keeps you from being active (or more active, or as active as you would like to be).

Develop a few creative solutions.

Evaluate your list of solutions. In the following space, write the solution you are willing to try and exactly *when* you will put it into action.

Analyze how well your plan worked and revise it if necessary. If your plan worked well, great! If your plan did not work too well, look back at your list of solutions and try again.

From B. Marcus and D. Pekmezi, *Motivating People to be Physically Active,* 3rd ed. (Champaign, IL: Human Kinetics, 2025). Adapted from S.N. Blair, A.L. Dunn, B.H. Marcus, et al., *Active Living Every Day,* 2nd ed. (Champaign, IL: Human Kinetics, 2011).

Develop a List of Solutions

Help your clients brainstorm and come up with as many creative solutions as possible. If they have trouble thinking up solutions, step in and offer some. Be sure to think broadly and to keep in mind what your client has already revealed about themselves. That is, try to personalize your responses as much as possible. Encourage them not to worry about whether any given solution is good or bad, workable or unrealistic. That can come later. Sometimes a client's seemingly far-fetched idea turns out to be the best solution. Have your clients write down all the ideas that come up and encourage them to keep the list with them for a few days so they can add more solutions as they think of them.

Evaluate the Solutions

Some solutions seem more realistic than others. However, solutions that seem far-fetched at first may appear more realistic with more thought. Work with your clients to select one solution they are willing to try. Then help them plan how and when to put it into action. For example, if your client's main barrier is not having a gym membership and the specific problem is not feeling safe walking in the community, one solution could involve teaching a simple aerobic exercise routine that can be done safely at home. Other plans might be to walk in the neighborhood with a partner or go to local parks or heavily traveled areas where it feels safe.

Analyze How Well the Plan Worked

After your client has given the plan a try, help analyze how well it worked. Help your client evaluate what did and did not work. Then tweak the plan as necessary. For example, if your client planned to rely on walking with a partner but never asked anyone, it is clear that the plan did not work because it was not implemented. Thus, there is no reason to throw this plan away; rather, your client should try it again. However, if your client asked family and friends to walk and they all declined, it might be necessary to revise the plan and perhaps try the home-based aerobic routine the next time. Because most clients have more than one barrier to address, you can encourage them to use the IDEA form for other barriers once they have used it successfully.

CONFIDENCE

Having confidence in oneself is critical during all phases of behavior change. Research in the psychology field has demonstrated that helping people believe in themselves and visualize themselves as people who are, or one day will

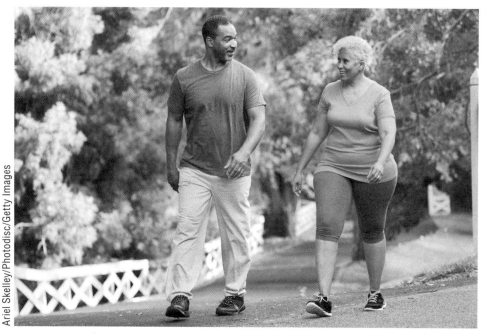

You and your client can come up with some innovative solutions to physical activity barriers using the IDEA approach.

be, successful is key to helping them think about change, make change, and sustain change over the years. You can help by regularly conveying your belief that your clients can and will succeed in their efforts to start or maintain a physical activity plan. Second, you can also teach your clients the skills to increase their belief in themselves, because this is critical once their contact with you has concluded.

To gauge your clients' level of confidence, ask them to rate their confidence that they can start being or continue to be regularly physically active on a scale of 1 to 5, with the lowest level of confidence being 1 and the highest level being 5. (For a more detailed questionnaire to measure confidence, see questionnaire 4.2 in appendix A.)

- If your clients answer 1 or 2, help them think about why they do not feel confident and discuss ways to help them become more confident. Pinpointing specific obstacles is often the first step to overcoming them. For example, if your client lacks confidence that exercising after work will succeed because of family responsibilities, you can suggest walking during breaks and lunchtime, and thus your client will have already accumulated 30 minutes of physical activity before going home.

- If your clients rate their confidence at 3, they are over halfway there. Help them think about what they like most and least about physical activity. Encourage the clients to do what they can to make physical activity more enjoyable, convenient, or safe for them. For example, ask whether your client prefers to be active alone or with others, and whether your client prefers to be active during the workday or before or after work. Try to determine the reason for these preferences. Perhaps your client prefers walking alone because of feelings of embarrassment about being too unfit to jog, an activity in which many friends participate. This may be important information if you learn that your client actually prefers being active with others and aspires to join friends eventually for early morning jogs.

- If your clients answered 4 or 5, they are well on their way to making exercise a lifelong habit. Maintaining a physically active lifestyle is extremely challenging. Staying active requires continued time, energy, and planning for a lifetime. To stay regularly active, a person needs to set the alarm clock to go off early in the morning, skip part of lunch to take a walk, or stop at the gym on the way home from work every day. Participating in physical activity never ceases to be an issue. Your clients may well begin to truly enjoy activity and even look forward to it. However, it always takes thought, time, and planning. Thus, it is critical that they remain confident that they can stick with physical activity even during times of stress, sadness, or extreme pressure at work. Work with them to instill the confidence that they can start their physical activity program anew if their efforts get derailed, such as following the birth of a child or relocating to a new city.

SET SHORT- AND LONG-TERM GOALS

Setting goals with your clients will help with their activity plan. The goals you set together become the contract you agree to pursue. The clearer the goals are, the better the chances of reaching them will be. Teaching your clients effective ways of setting goals can be instrumental in helping them succeed. *It is important to set both short-term and long-term goals.* If your client's long-term goal is to walk 30 minutes a day, five days a week, the client should not expect to reach that goal immediately. Help the client recognize the need to start off slowly yet never lose sight of the goal. A good short-term goal might be to walk for 10 minutes on Sunday, Wednesday, and Friday, then gradually increase the number of minutes and the number of days a week of walking. In this way, clients build confidence that they can meet their goals, which will then empower them to set future goals. Reaching one's goal creates a sense of mastery and a warm sense of achievement. Figure 7.6 is an example of a form you and your client can use to record goals. Give your clients feedback, and teach them to give themselves feedback. Choose a way to track your clients' progress. Chapters 2, 4, and 6 suggest assessment tools. Monitoring progress lets your clients see the pattern of ups and downs and helps them understand that the downs are only temporary. They can then learn strategies to turn these downs into ups and to avoid some of these downs in the future.

Figure 7.6 Goal-setting form.

My short-term goal that I plan to achieve next week:
How I plan to monitor my progress on reaching this goal:
My long-term goal I plan to achieve by _____ (date):
How I plan to monitor my progress on reaching this goal:

From B. Marcus and D. Pekmezi, *Motivating People to be Physically Active,* 3rd ed. (Champaign, IL: Human Kinetics, 2025). Adapted from S.N. Blair, A.L. Dunn, B.H. Marcus, et al., *Active Living Every Day,* 2nd ed. (Champaign, IL: Human Kinetics, 2011).

LEARNING HOW IT WORKS
How to Select SMART Goals

When selecting goals, be sure they are SMART (specific, measurable, achievable, realistic, and time bound; figure 7.7; Doran, 1981).

- *Specific:* People who set specific goals do better than people who say, "I'll try to do my best." For example, if your clients say, "I will try to be more active," help them turn this into a more specific goal (e.g., specify the preferred activity), "I will try to walk more this week." You can even discuss where this walk will occur (at the park) and who will join them on this walk (a neighbor). Specific goals tend to be more effective.
- *Measurable:* It is hard to judge success with goals like "I will try to walk more this week." Tracking one's progress (recording the time spent walking) and selecting quantifiable metrics for success are key (10 minutes). For example, "I will try to take an extra 10-minute walk this week." Progress toward such a goal can be easily monitored, and thus one's achievement is clear.
- *Achievable and Realistic:* With your assistance, your clients can set specific goals that they can realistically attain. For example, if your client is rather sedentary and has no experience with or affinity for running, goals related to a brief walking bout will be more appropriate than attacking a 5-kilometer run. Goal setting is related to confidence building; if your client reaches a goal (e.g., the 10-minute walk), your client will have increased confidence in progressing to meet the next goal. Success breeds success.
- *Time bound:* Good goals should include clear plans and deadlines. For example, the goal "I will try to take an extra 10-minute walk this week," does not state when the actual walk will occur. Success may be more likely if the client reviews the calendar and designates a specific date and time for the walk. "I will try to take a 10-minute walk at 5 p.m. on Wednesday."

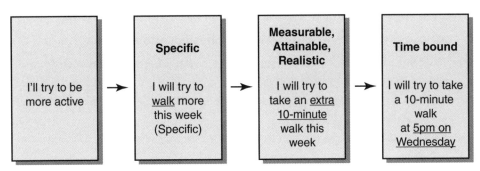

Figure 7.7 SMART goals example.

MEASURE SUCCESS

There are several ways to measure success in physical activity. You can encourage your clients to track their physical activity (e.g., step counts, time spent exercising) and set a goal (e.g., increasing their step count, activity time). You can also use any of the questionnaires in appendix A, re-administering them every three months to evaluate your clients' progress. You and your clients can also evaluate the new strategies they have learned and other strategies that may be helpful in their movement toward becoming more physically active.

Goal setting is valuable only when you can measure success in attaining goals. For your clients to feel successful, you and your client must agree on what constitutes success. At different points, you may measure success by different means. Initially, success may be measured more by changes in the mediators of change in physical activity described in chapter 4. Later, success may be measured by forward progression in the stages of change as described in chapter 2 or by changes in fitness as described in chapter 6. Measuring success is important for keeping your clients on track and ensuring that short- and long-term goals stay realistic.

The following sidebar illustrates how to use the information presented in this chapter to help a client become more active. The process of becoming more active is not always smooth; it often requires repeated problem-solving and patience.

> ### Stage-Specific Strategies for Individual Counseling
>
> This section provides strategies to use in individual counseling with clients. They are broken down into stages of readiness for change.

Stage 1: Not Thinking About Change

Even though your client is not considering becoming physically active right now, you can still do some brief counseling to help your client move toward thinking about behavior change. Here are some ways you can apply the strategies discussed in this chapter for a client at this earliest stage.

Is your client physically ready to begin physical activity?

- Give your client the PAR-Q (figure 7.1) to identify any health reasons that would preclude physical activity.
- Explain to your client that moderate-intensity activity is unlikely to cause adverse health events.
- Refer your client to a physician if any health problems exist.

How has your client successfully changed behavior in the past?

- Increase your client's confidence by discussing any past attempts at behavior change and identifying strategies that worked then and could help with physical activity change in the future (figure 7.2).
- Address any problems that have gotten in your client's way during past attempts at behavior change (figure 7.5).

How might your client benefit from physical activity?

- Ask your client to write about the possible benefits of some physical activity (figure 7.3).
- Suggest some benefits your client may not have thought of yet.
- Encourage your client to learn more about the benefits of physical activity.
- Have your client assess how important these benefits are.

What might your client need to give up to become physically active, and what barriers does your client need to address?

- Ask your client to write down what would have to be given up to become physically active and what might be unpleasant about physical activity (figure 7.4).

What goals might help your client move toward behavior change?

- Work with your client to set a manageable, short-term goal, perhaps around a mediator of behavior change (see chapter 4) that can help your client start thinking about a lifestyle change (figure 7.6).
- Ask your client to discuss with the physician the possible benefits of some physical activity (comprehending benefits; figure 7.5).
- Ask your client to try to identify a similar person in age, body shape, and health status who is being physically active (self-efficacy).
- Have your client ask a friend or family member to take over childcare or household responsibilities for an hour so that your client can take a tour of the local YMCA (enlisting social support, increasing knowledge).
- Ask your client to write down some ways that a sedentary lifestyle is affecting people important to them (caring about consequences to others).
- Reinforce any action your client takes that helps in thinking about trying some physical activity (e.g., talking to others about physical activity, reading about it, thinking about the possible benefits of becoming physically active).

How can you measure your client's success?

- Reassess your client's stage of change (see chapter 2).
- Consider giving your client the processes of change questionnaire (questionnaire 4.1 in appendix A) to see whether your client is using more strategies.

- Measure your client's confidence to see whether it has improved, using the self-efficacy questionnaire (questionnaire 4.2 in appendix A).
- Reassess your client's perceived benefits relative to the perceived barriers using the decisional balance questionnaire (questionnaire 4.4 in appendix A).
- Ask your client to simply rate satisfaction with the progress on a scale of 1 to 5.

Stage 2: Thinking About Change

Your client is thinking about becoming more active, so your task is to help your client commit to a start date and do some planning that will enhance the likelihood of success in this endeavor and find the physical activity experience pleasant enough to try it again. Here are some ideas for helping a client who is thinking about change but has not yet engaged in any actual physical activity.

Is your client physically ready to begin physical activity?

- Give your client the PAR-Q (figure 7.1) to identify any health reasons that would preclude physical activity.
- Explain to your client that moderate-intensity activity is unlikely to cause adverse health events.
- Refer your client to a physician if any health problems exist or if your client expresses interest in starting with vigorous activity.

How has your client successfully changed behavior in the past?

- Increase your client's self-efficacy by discussing past attempts at behavior change and identifying strategies that worked then and could help with beginning physical activity now (figure 7.2).
- Address any problems that have gotten in the way during past attempts at behavior change and may become an issue for changing physical activity habits (figure 7.5).

How might your client benefit from physical activity?

- Ask your client to write about the possible benefits of physical activity (figure 7.3).
- Suggest some benefits your client may not have thought of yet.
- Encourage your client to learn more about the benefits of physical activity.
- Have your client assess how important these benefits are.

What might your client need to give up to become physically active, and what barriers does your client need to address?

- Ask your client to write down what would have to be given up to become physically active and what might be unpleasant about physical activity (figure 7.4).

- Have your client assess how important these issues are.
- Help your client find solutions to these barriers using the IDEA approach (figure 7.5).

How can you help your client become more confident about physical activity?

- Let your client know that you believe in their ability to become a physically active person.
- Emphasize that your client has already made progress by thinking about becoming physically active.
- Work on increasing your client's confidence by trying to pinpoint perceived obstacles and developing realistic strategies for overcoming them (figures 7.4 and 7.5).
- Relate your client's past successes at behavior change with the ability to become physically active in the future (figure 7.2).
- Discuss what went wrong during past attempts at behavior change and reframe them as learning experiences that can teach your client what to do differently when deciding to become physically active.
- Begin to identify types of activities that might be manageable and enjoyable for your client to try. Plan when, where, and with whom your client might do these activities so they can be clearly visualized.

What goals might help your client move toward behavior change?

- Work with your client to set manageable short- and long-term goals, perhaps around a mediator of behavior change (see chapter 4) that can help to move closer to actually trying some physical activity (figure 7.6).
- Recommend that your client make a few calls to learn where the chosen activity might be performed (increasing knowledge).
- Ask your client to try the IDEA approach (figure 7.5) to work out solutions to one or two of the obstacles that seem to get in the way of actually trying some activity (decisional balance).
- Recommend that your client ask someone with whom they are close to help address some of the barriers that have been identified (enlisting social support).
- Suggest that your client commit to actually trying a brief, manageable bout of physical activity, such as a five-minute walk (self-efficacy, committing oneself).
- Ask your client to complete a personal time study like that found in chapter 6 (e.g., monitoring time spent in sedentary pursuits and in physical activity for a typical weekday and weekend day, increasing knowledge).
- Ask your client to write down some ways that a sedentary lifestyle is affecting people important to them (caring about consequences to others).

Has your client been successful in moving toward becoming physically active?

- Reassess your client's stage of change (see chapter 2).
- Consider giving your client the processes of change questionnaire (questionnaire 4.1 in appendix A).
- Measure your client's confidence by using the self-efficacy questionnaire (questionnaire 4.2 in appendix A) to see whether it has improved.
- Reassess your client's perceived benefits relative to perceived barriers using the decisional balance questionnaire (questionnaire 4.4 in appendix A).
- Ask your client to simply rate satisfaction with the progress on a scale of 1 to 5.

Stage 3: Doing Some Physical Activity

Your client is doing some physical activity but is not meeting public health guidelines yet. Your client would like help developing some additional strategies for increasing activity levels. Here are some ideas for a client in this stage.

Is your client physically ready to increase physical activity?

- Give your client the PAR-Q (figure 7.1) to identify any health reasons that would preclude physical activity.
- Explain to your client that moderate-intensity activity is unlikely to cause adverse health events.
- Refer your client to a physician if any health problems exist.

How has your client changed behavior in the past?

- Increase your client's self-efficacy by discussing past attempts at behavior change and identifying strategies that worked then and could help with increasing physical activity now (figure 7.2).
- Address any problems that have gotten in the way during past attempts at behavior change and may become an issue for changing physical activity now (figure 7.5).

How might your client benefit from increasing physical activity?

- Ask your client to write about the possible benefits of increasing physical activity (figure 7.3).
- Suggest some benefits your client may not have thought of yet or has not yet noticed. Encourage your client to learn more about these benefits and to look for additional benefits from increasing physical activity.
- Have your client assess how important these benefits are.

What might your client need to give up to become more physically active, and what barriers does your client need to address?

- Ask your client to write down what would have to be given up to increase physical activity and what might be unpleasant about physical activity (figure 7.4).
- Have your client assess how difficult these things will be to give up.
- Help your client find solutions for these barriers using the IDEA approach (figure 7.5).

How can you help your client become more confident about physical activity?

- Let your client know that you believe in their ability to increase physical activity.
- Emphasize that your client has already made progress by doing some physical activity.
- Work on increasing your client's confidence by pinpointing perceived obstacles and developing realistic strategies for overcoming them (figures 7.4 and 7.5).
- Relate your client's past successes at behavior change with the ability to become more physically active (figure 7.2).
- Discuss what went wrong during past attempts at behavior change and reframe them as learning experiences that can teach your client what to do differently this time.
- Help your client think about what they like most and least about physical activity and how the activity plans can be modified to reflect these preferences.
- Encourage your client to think of themselves as a physically active person.

What goals might help your client become more physically active?

- Work with your client to set manageable short- and long-term goals, perhaps around a mediator of behavior change (see chapter 4) that can help your client increase physical activity (figure 7.6).
- Create a plan for replacing 15 minutes of sedentary time during the week with some type of activity (substituting alternatives).
- Suggest that your client set a goal of asking a friend to join a 20-minute walk in the upcoming week (enlisting social support).
- Help your client think of a couple of reminders to be more active and suggest trying to implement them over the week (reminding oneself).
- Encourage your client to commit to increasing daily activity by five more minutes over the next week (self-efficacy, committing oneself).
- Agree on something nice your client can do (e.g., visit a farmers' market, pick up a new book at the library) as a reward for achieving the goal/s (rewarding oneself).

- Set up a point system that your client can use to earn a larger reward (e.g., accomplishing a small goal earns 2 points; 30 accumulated points can purchase a new yoga mat).
- Discuss what someone significant in your client's life might do or say to reward your client's physical activity achievements (enlisting social support).

Has your client succeeded in increasing physical activity?

- Have your client wear an activity tracker (e.g., pedometer, wristband, or smartwatch) or keep a daily activity log to monitor minutes of activity (figure 6.2).
- Ask your client to write down the number of steps accumulated on a step counter over the course of the day (figures 6.5).
- Reassess your client's stage of change (see chapter 2).
- Consider giving your client the processes of change questionnaire (questionnaire 4.1 in appendix A) to see whether your client is using more strategies for change.
- Measure your client's confidence to see whether it has improved by using the self-efficacy questionnaire (questionnaire 4.2 in appendix A).
- Administer the decisional balance questionnaire (questionnaire 4.4 in appendix A).

Stage 4: Doing Enough Physical Activity

Even though your client is physically active at the recommended level, the challenge is to maintain physical activity over time. Here are some suggestions for using the strategies discussed in this chapter to help a client in this stage make physical activity a habit.

Is it physically safe for your client to continue being physically active?

- Give your client the PAR-Q (figure 7.1) to assess any changes in health status relevant to physical activity.
- Refer your client to a physician if any health problems or discomforts related to activity arise.

How has your client changed behavior in the past?

- Discuss your client's past attempts at behavior change to identify strategies that may not have been applied yet to physical activity (figure 7.2).
- Address any problems that have gotten in the way during past attempts at behavior change and may be an issue for continuing physical activity (figure 7.5).

How has your client benefited from becoming physically active?

- Ask your client to write about the benefits of physical activity (figure 7.3).
- Suggest some benefits your client may not have thought of yet or has not yet noticed.
- Encourage your client to learn more about the benefits of physical activity and to look for additional benefits from continuing to be physically active.
- Have your client assess how important these benefits are.

What are the costs of being physically active? What barriers might your client still need to address?

- Ask your client to write down what has been given up to become physically active and what is still unpleasant about physical activity (figure 7.4).
- Have your client assess how important these things are.
- Use the IDEA problem-solving approach to reduce any perceived costs and any remaining barriers (figure 7.5).
- Encourage your client to think about any obstacles that might arise in the future that could interfere with staying active. Create a plan for these potential problems.

How can your client become even more confident about physical activity?

- Discuss any negative thoughts concerning physical activity with which your client is still struggling and work on developing more positive thoughts.
- Help your client think about what they like most and least about physical activity. Discover what you can do to help make physical activity more enjoyable, convenient, or safe for your client.
- Work with your client to instill confidence in starting the physical activity program anew, if for some reason it is stopped.
- Remind your client of how far they have come and praise their efforts.

What goals might help your client stay physically active?

- Help your client generate short-term goals for physical activity or for mediators that may help sustain motivation.
- Help your client decide on an appropriate amount of activity in a given week (committing oneself).
- Suggest that your client try a new activity (enjoyment).
- Encourage your client to ask someone to be an exercise partner (enlisting social support).
- Suggest that your client think of someone for whom they can serve as an exercise role model. Have your client commit to a behavior that might help motivate this person to become active (caring about consequences to others, committing oneself).

- Help your client develop some long-term goals (committing oneself; see figure 7.6).
- Find a walking, biking, running event, or race that is going to take place in the community. Work on a plan for your client to participate (committing oneself).
- Set up a reward plan for your client's continued regular activity for the next month (rewarding oneself).
- Help your client decide on a number of miles to try to accumulate over the next three months (goal setting).
- Consult with a health professional, if necessary, to determine appropriate physiological goals for your client, such as decreasing cholesterol or blood pressure.
- Agree on a small gift your client can buy for accomplishing the goal (rewarding oneself).
- Suggest that your client engage in a pleasurable activity (e.g., watching a favorite movie, reading a magazine, taking a short nap) after accomplishing one activity goal.
- Set up a point system that your client can use to earn a larger reward (e.g., accomplishing a small goal earns 2 points; 50 accumulated points can be used toward a game night with friends or family).
- Discuss what someone significant in your client's life might do or say to reward your client's physical activity achievements (enlisting social support).
- Remind your client to review some benefits that have already been achieved from physical activity. These benefits are natural rewards for exercising.
- Suggest that your clients post some reminders in the environment to praise themselves for success (reminding oneself).

How can your client track success?

- Have your client keep a daily activity log to monitor minutes of activity (figure 6.2).
- Ask your client to track the number of steps accumulated on a step counter over the course of the day (see chapter 6) or track this information via a wristband and smart phone app. Develop a reward plan for your client after achieving a particular number.
- Suggest that your client monitor the resting heart rate and level of exertion during activity. Have your client record them on a graph (or track them via a smart phone app) to see the changes over time.
- If your client has a short period of inactivity (because of work demands or illness) but then resumes activity following this episode, praise your client for getting back on track.

Stage 5: Making Physical Activity a Habit

Your client is somewhat of a seasoned pro in this stage. However, you can be beneficial by using the strategies discussed in this chapter to help your client prepare for any future setbacks and increase your client's enjoyment of physical activity.

Is it physically safe for your client to continue being physically active?

- Give your client the PAR-Q (figure 7.1) to assess any changes in health status relevant to physical activity.
- Refer your client to a physician if any health problems arise.

How has your client changed behavior in the past?

- Discuss your client's past attempts at behavior change to identify strategies that may not have been applied yet to physical activity.
- Address any problems that have gotten in the way during past attempts at behavior change and may be an issue for continuing physical activity (figure 7.5).

How has your client benefited from continuing to be physically active?

- Suggest some benefits from physical activity that your client may not have noticed.
- Encourage your client to learn more about the benefits of physical activity.
- Encourage your client to periodically remind themselves of the benefits of continuing to be physically active; this helps to sustain motivation (figure 7.3).

What are the costs of being physically active? What barriers might your client still need to address?

- Ask your client to write down what has been given up to become physically active and what is still unpleasant about physical activity (figure 7.4).
- Have your client assess how important these things are.
- Use the IDEA problem-solving approach to further reduce any perceived costs (figure 7.5).
- Work with your client to come up with ways to increase the enjoyment of physical activity.
- Encourage your client to think about any obstacles that might arise in the future and interfere with staying active. Help your client create a plan for these potential problems.

How can your client maintain confidence about staying active over the long term?

- Explore with your client options for making activity more enjoyable.
- Work with your client to instill confidence in starting the physical activity program anew, if for some reason it is stopped.
- Remind your client of how far they have come and praise their efforts.
- Remind your client of the benefits already achieved.
- Encourage your client to become a mentor to someone else who is trying to accomplish what your client already has.

What goals might help your client stay physically active?

- Help your client generate short-term goals to sustain motivation (committing oneself; see figure 7.6).
- Suggest that your client try a new activity (enjoyment).
- Encourage your client to ask someone to be a physical activity partner (enlisting social support).
- Suggest that your client think of someone for whom they can serve as an exercise role model. Have your client commit to a behavior that might help motivate this person to become active (caring about consequences to others, committing oneself).
- Help your client develop some long-term goals (committing oneself).
- Find a walking, biking, or running event that is going to take place in the community. Work on a plan for your client to prepare for this event (committing oneself).
- Set up a reward plan for your client's continued regular activity for the next month (rewarding oneself).
- Help your client decide on a number of miles to try to accumulate over the next three months (goal setting). For example, your client could set a challenge to reach 30 miles (48.3 km) per month.
- Consult with a health professional, if necessary, to determine appropriate physiological goals for your client, such as decreasing cholesterol or blood pressure.
- Agree on something nice your client can do when the goal is accomplished (rewarding oneself).
- Suggest that your client engage in some pleasurable activity (e.g., talking to a friend on the phone) after accomplishing one activity goal.
- Set up a point system that your client can use to earn a larger reward (e.g., accomplishing a small goal earns 2 points; 80 accumulated points can purchase a new water bottle).
- Discuss what someone significant in your client's life might do or say as a reward for physical activity achievements (enlisting social support).

- Remind your client to look over some benefits already achieved from physical activity. These benefits are natural rewards for exercising.
- Suggest that your clients post some reminders in the environment to remember to praise themselves for success (reminding oneself).

How can your client track success?

- Have your client keep a daily activity log to monitor minutes of activity (see figure 6.2).
- Ask your client to track the number of steps each day using a pedometer (see figure 6.5; e.g., a wristband or smartphone app).
- Help your client develop a reward plan for achieving a particular number.
- Suggest that your client monitor the resting heart rate (figure 6.6) and level of exertion during activity. Have your client record these on a graph (use an app to track them) to see the changes over time.
- If your client has a short period of inactivity (because of work demands or illness) but then resumes activity following this episode, praise your client for getting back on track.

CASE EXAMPLE

CREATING CHANGE THROUGH INDIVIDUAL COUNSELING

Rose, a 28-year-old single mother, was referred for physical activity counseling by her primary care physician. She had a lifelong history of obesity and knew that managing her weight and lowering her blood pressure would require that she make some changes. She agreed to seek physical activity counseling.

At the beginning, Rose completed a physical activity history questionnaire (see questionnaire 7.1) and the physical activity stages of change questionnaire (see questionnaire 2.1). Her responses on these assessments indicated that she had never been physically active for any significant amount of time, but she was in stage 2 (thinking about change). Other measures identified low self-efficacy for physical activity and several barriers that prevented her from being physically active (e.g., low energy, little time, physical discomfort, difficulty finding enjoyable activities). Moreover, Rose scored low on the processes of change questionnaire, indicating that she had made few steps toward becoming more active to date.

To boost her motivation, Rose was encouraged to focus on what she had to gain by becoming more active, such as improved health, increased energy, and setting a positive example for her five-year-old son. To build her confidence, Rose reflected on past successful behavior changes (e.g., drinking more water) and how this was accomplished. Rose recalled setting small goals (drinking one or two glasses of water with meals, then sipping on water while at her desk), making environmental changes (keeping a water bottle handy and

(continued)

Creating Change Through Individual Counseling *(continued)*

no soda in her house), and creating reminders (placing sticky notes on her refrigerator and computer). Rose developed a plan for using similar strategies for physical activity. She set a modest weekly goal of three 15-minute walks around the block and put her walking shoes by the door as a reminder. She was concerned about childcare, but using the IDEA approach, she came up with the solution of having her son ride his bicycle beside her while she walked. Rose was excited and felt like she could do this.

However, two weeks later, Rose admitted that an unexpected cold snap interfered with her goal of walking outside. She used the IDEA approach to brainstorm how to be active inside when the weather is inclement. Rose mentioned that her mother had a treadmill that she might use. Rose decided to ask to use her mother's treadmill and met the goal of three 15-minute walks a week.

A few weeks later, Rosemary again admitted that she had not met her physical activity goal. She kept meaning to go over to her mother's house to use the treadmill after work, but she just never got around to it. At this point Rose reviewed what she had to gain by increasing her physical activity and considered how to complete her activity goal during the day before she got home and needed to take care of her son and the house.

Although her workplace had an exercise facility for employees, Rose felt self-conscious about her size and did not want to exercise in such a public place. She also decided against using her lunch break for taking a walk because that was when she ran errands that she did not think she would otherwise get done. However, Rose agreed that a good way to start might be to use the stairs to get to her third-floor office (rather than the elevator) three times each workday. This would not take too much time or involve a big audience and would be a step in the right direction.

Rose reported good news a few weeks later. She had met her goal of using the stairs three times daily and felt encouraged enough to try doing this at the doctor's office and at the mall. Although she was still far from the 60 minutes of daily moderate-intensity activity that was her ultimate goal, this success helped move her to stage 3 (doing some physical activity) and boosted her self-efficacy. Over the course of the next six months, she was able to incorporate other activities such as a weekly game of tag with her son, gardening on the weekends, and taking a walk outdoors at least once a week. She set up rewards for making progress toward her goals (e.g., watching her favorite movie). She was well on her way to developing a physically active lifestyle.

INDIVIDUAL COUNSELING AND REMOTE TECHNOLOGIES

Individual counseling is often provided face-to-face by a live health coach in a clinic. In fact, this has been considered the gold standard of practice until recently. Yet, times are changing, and numerous convenient remote strategies are now available. Individual counseling can occur via telephone, text messaging, websites, and smart phone applications, among other technologies. Video conferencing became common practice for many during the COVID-19 pandemic and allows for particularly engaging interpersonal interactions without requiring transportation, childcare, or other barriers to meeting. Finally, individual physical activity does not necessarily have to be provided in real time by health coaches. Physical activity counseling calls and text messages can now be easily automated (using tailoring algorithms, message banks, communication application programming interfaces, and software) for greater reach and reduced costs.

CONCLUSION

In this chapter we showed how the stages of change model can be applied to working with individuals. We shared the rationale and tools for assessing your client's physical and psychological readiness for physical activity. The PAR-Q was provided as an example of an instrument used to screen clients for medical concerns and determine whether physical activity can be safely increased. We also described the importance of discussing your client's experiences in making behavior changes and how this information can guide current plans for behavior change. Specific strategies for measuring your client's confidence, weighing the pros and cons of behavior change, problem-solving (IDEA), and goal setting (SMART) were described. We also discussed the need to measure change in your client's behavior to empower your client to continue the journey of behavior change and the maintenance of that change. Examples of strategies to use in individual counseling with clients were shared for each of the 5 stages of motivational readiness for physical activity. Finally, we acknowledged how innovative technologies can be used to provide individual physical activity counseling to more people (in the comfort of their homes) at lower costs.

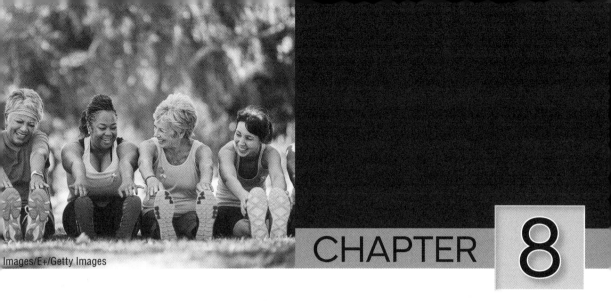
Images/E+/Getty Images

CHAPTER 8

Using the Stages Model in Group Counseling Programs

Group counseling can be a cost- and time-effective way for health promoters to help several people at once. Research shows that group therapy is sometimes even more beneficial than individual therapy (Pappas, 2023). A group-based physical activity program can offer participants additional ideas about becoming more active through other group members' experiences and thoughts on the subject. Group physical activity programs provide additional channels of social support through relationships with group members and the group leader. Group members may choose to get together and communicate outside of the regular group meetings and thus provide each other with more regular support. The group leader can facilitate this by encouraging group members to connect and call upon each other during tough times or for problem-solving and support.

Group programs can be offered virtually via social media, smart phone applications, and video conferencing, with similar outcomes as in-person groups (Gentry et al., 2019). A recent study in which participants used an interactive online physical activity tracking platform (Walk Georgia) as individuals or groups found that group users logged more minutes of physical activity and met national physical activity guidelines on more weeks than individual users (Smith et al., 2018). Clients can further develop online support by posting about their physical activity challenges and successes and reacting and commenting on discussion threads or schedules.

Many types of groups promote physical activity. People engaging in physical activity in the same place (e.g., gym or pool) or at the same time (e.g., via live video-delivered group walking sessions; Browne et al., 2023), and an instructor leading a group of people in an exercise class can all be considered group-based programs. Other groups may provide health education and specific skill-building strategies and behavioral techniques that apply psychological theory to behavior change. Whether you develop a health education group, a behavioral skill-building group, or group exercise classes (or some combination thereof) will depend on the setting, your professional training, and the needs and interests of your clients. Our purpose in this chapter is to discuss strategies for incorporating the stages of motivational readiness for change model in group programs that teach members behavioral skills to help incorporate physical activity into their daily lives.

LEADING A STAGE-BASED GROUP

Group programs are influenced by group members' stages of motivational readiness for change and by the role and teaching style of the group leader (Rinne & Toropainen, 1998). You are likely to adopt the role of *teacher* and use a didactic leadership style more often with clients who are in the earlier stages of motivational readiness (stage 1, not thinking about change, and stage 2, thinking about change). For clients in stage 2, thinking about change, and stage 3, doing some physical activity, you may find yourself being a *motivator* who encourages them to try new skills. For clients in stages 3 (doing some activity) and 4 (doing moderate activity), you can also be less didactic and serve more as a *facilitator*, who encourages group members to share ideas, experiences, and support. For clients in the later stages, 4 and 5 (doing enough physical activity and making physical activity a habit, respectively), you will probably find that you need to give even less information but rather serve as an *analyzer*, who helps clients identify potential pitfalls, and as a *consultant*, who offers suggestions for avoiding pitfalls or handling them better. As the group leader, you will also need to be flexible about your role and instructional style when the people in your group are at different stages of motivational readiness for change (Rinne & Toropainen, 1998). Table 8.1 describes teaching styles and instructor roles suited to each of the stages of motivational readiness.

Table 8.1 Group Leader's Role and Teaching Style in a Stage-Based Group

Stage	Leader's role	Teaching style	Sample input
1: Not thinking about change	Teacher	Share information	"Here are some physical and mental health benefits to physical activity."
2: Thinking about change	Teacher Motivator	Share information Provide encouragement, increase confidence	"Research studies have shown that even small bouts of physical activity are good for you. Every movement counts!" "Getting started can be as easy as taking a stroll to the mailbox. Keep it simple at first! You got this."

Stage	Leader's role	Teaching style	Sample input
3: Doing some activity	Teacher Motivator Facilitator	Share information Provide encouragement Promote group process (e.g., sharing of ideas and support amongst group members)	"If you want to be more active, it is important to track your daily physical activity and reward yourself for making progress. I will share some strategies for how to do this." "Look at those extra steps this week. Way to go! Be sure to do something nice for yourself for meeting this goal." "How do you fit physical activity into a busy day?"
4: Doing enough activity	Facilitator Analyzer Consultant	Promote group process Help identify potential hazards Propose relapse prevention strategies (e.g., avoiding slips, better handling of barriers)	"Sometimes we don't feel like being active. We may need a pep talk to get going. What could we tell ourselves for motivation?" "You have spent a lot of time walking at the park lately. But it is about to get hot. What is the plan for staying active this summer?" "When you get busy, physical activity sometimes falls off the radar. Getting a workout in before the day gets hectic might help you stick with it. Let's discuss scheduling physical activity for first thing in the morning and how that might work for you."
5: Making activity a habit	Motivator Facilitator Analyzer Consultant	Provide encouragement Promote group process Help identify potential pitfalls Suggest strategies for preventing relapse	"You have been regularly physically active for over 6 months. That is fantastic!" "Why don't we all share helpful tips for staying active over the long term? What strategies have worked best for you?" "What is the trick to staying active? Many people will say enjoying it. People tend to quit when they are no longer having fun. Let's talk about ways to keep physical activity enjoyable and avoid boredom." "Sometimes life happens, and we stop being active for a while. Things tend to come up (illness, injury, etc.). How will you get back on track with exercise after an exercise break? Let's make a plan."

Adapted from Rinne and Toropainen (1998).

LEARNING HOW IT WORKS
Promoting Social Support While Leading Physical Activity Group Counseling Sessions

Group-based physical activity programs provide wonderful opportunities for enhancing social support for lifestyle change. As a leader, you can provide social support both directly (through your relationships with participants) and indirectly (by encouraging participants to connect with each other and designing and implementing activities to help them reflect on and address social support needs). But how?

A recent study shed light on how instructors influence social support (particularly among older adults) in physical activity group settings. After conducting observations of 16 group physical activity classes, focus groups, and interviews ($N=38$) with the class participants (Morrison et al., 2023), several themes emerged related to how the instructors provided social support (e.g., by developing caring relationships, establishing a welcoming environment, and managing conflict). Here are some tips on how to achieve these goals in your groups.

Before group

- Consider creating physical activity groups based on common experiences, interests, and health concerns (e.g., a group for new mothers, individuals with type 2 diabetes, etc.). This will help group members relate to one another and support each other.
- Develop group guidelines by making ground rules for group participation (i.e., members will use respectful language, etc.) and strategies for handling any potential violations (name-calling may result in being asked to leave).
- Request that "what is said in group stays in group." While there are always limits to confidentiality in group settings, such reminders help participants understand appropriate group etiquette upfront and make everyone feel a bit more comfortable sharing.

During group

- Start each session with greetings and introductions (as needed).
- Check in on individual progress toward goals.
- Listen reflectively. (Summarize what participants said in your own words: "It sounds like you had a tough week.")
- Praise any wins. ("Way to go for fitting that walk into your lunch break!")
- Respond with empathy when participants describe challenges. ("I am sorry your son was sick. I bet that did make it hard to exercise yesterday.")
- Make eye contact with group members. (Remember to look into the web camera if meeting virtually.)

- Use body language and hand gestures to help express your ideas.
- Encourage all group members to contribute to the conversation. (Ask questions of the group, allow each member time to answer, encourage quieter participants to speak up, and discourage one or two members from monopolizing the conversation.)
- Facilitate interactions among group members (breakout sessions, paired discussions).

Adapted from Health Resources & Services Administration, "Telehealth for Behavioral Health Care," last modified December 7, 2022, https://telehealth.hhs.gov/providers/best-practice-guides/telehealth-for-behavioral-health/group-teletherapy.

Setting Up a Stage-Based Group

There are no hard-and-fast rules about the number of people you should have in a group, how the counseling should be delivered, or the number of sessions you should hold. Groups with fewer members offer more opportunity for participation and instructor attention. Larger groups, on the other hand, are more cost and time effective. Both issues are important to consider when deciding the size of a group. Our general guideline is to have a maximum of 12 people if there is to be individual participation. Five people is probably the minimum useful number for idea sharing and discussions among the participants. That way, if one or two people cannot attend a given session, enough members will still be present to exchange thoughts and ideas.

Rinne and Toropainen (1998) suggested that two or three group sessions are not likely to have much impact, whereas group sessions that stretch over several months may become boring. For group treatment, 10 to 12 weekly group sessions are appropriate. If the group expresses an interest in continuing to meet, consider having a break at the end of 12 weeks or so and then scheduling a follow-up group in one month so that members can share their experiences of continuing their activity plans on their own (Rinne & Toropainen, 1998).

If you will be leading a larger group, consider having a colleague serve as a co-leader. It is always nice to have more than one professional perspective and to share the work of preparing for group and facilitating group discussions. If group members are in various stages of motivational readiness and you decide to break them up into smaller groups based on stage, each co-leader can take responsibility for facilitating a subgroup.

Consider calling participants who do not show up (or comment and engage) for a group session or two. Giving no-shows a quick call helps with accountability and lets them know that you missed their presence and perspective in the group. It also gives you a chance to learn whether something about the group made them decide not to participate or whether personal circumstances kept them from coming. Sometimes people drop out because they believe they are not making progress. A quick phone call to these people gives you an opportunity to reiterate that people's stages of readiness to make a personal behavior change vary and that attending group sessions should be considered progress in itself. You could also encourage the client to consider one or two individual sessions, if available, to get back on track before, or in addition to, rejoining the group. Whatever your policy is on missed sessions, tell the people in your group what it is at the outset so that they know what to expect.

LEARNING HOW IT WORKS
Conducting Physical Activity Group Counseling Sessions in a Virtual Environment

While most of the previously discussed logistics for leading in-person groups also apply when conducting groups remotely, there are some additional considerations. Thus, in this section, we will outline several tips and best practices for leading physical activity group counseling sessions in a virtual environment.

First, there is the matter of selecting which channel and what type of interaction (real time, asynchronous, or mixed) to provide. Group sessions can be held over live video conferencing calls, allowing group members to interact in real time. These live chats are popular, engaging remote approaches, but may be difficult for some participants to fit into their schedules. Asynchronous communication options are also available. Participants can interact through group email, web chat, or social media, among other methods. While there may be a time lag in communications, such forums allow participants to share experiences and respond to other members at their convenience. Many online applications provide opportunities for both real time and asynchronous group interactions.

Another practical consideration for virtual sessions is group size. If asynchronous participation is an option, larger numbers of participants might be appropriate and conducive to lively discussion threads, especially since some members may "lurk" without commenting or reacting. On the other hand, smaller numbers might be more appropriate for remote group counseling in real time to avoid clients speaking over each other.

Next, there is the matter of selecting virtual group settings for privacy, user controls, and more. Carefully consider which options you will use. For example, you may wish to set password and waiting room functions for sessions rather than allowing less controlled access. This can reduce the chances of uninvited guests attending the virtual group. Chat functions can be disabled to minimize side conversations during the session. Finally, consider setting screen sharing to "host only" to avoid inappropriate and unsolicited images or videos being shared in group.

You should also reflect on the additional confidentiality concerns for virtual versus in-person groups and review this information with participants. For example, virtual group members could make mistakes, such as logging into sessions from a public area, taking a screenshot, or recording during sessions. Ground rules for virtual groups usually include keeping the camera on during sessions; however, if individuals are concerned about privacy, the group leader can consider allowing participants to take precautions such as turning off web cams, participating using audio only, displaying avatars or using filters to disguise identity, and providing just first names or even fake names for on-screen identification.

While guidelines are critical for all groups, here are some tips specific to setting guidelines for virtual settings. Group leaders should ask participants to

- find a private space free of distractions for the session;
- place a "do not disturb" sign on the door and remind those nearby not to interrupt the session;
- attend the session alone and not allow non-members (e.g., family members) to listen to or watch the session;
- wear headphones or keep the volume low to prevent sound traveling;
- not record or take screenshots during group sessions;
- mute themselves when not speaking;
- use the "raise hand" feature (or physically raise their hand on camera) when they want to speak;
- use a secure internet connection, not public or free Wi-Fi;
- keep the webcam steady and at eye contact level; and
- place phones or computers in Airplane Mode to avoid interruptions.

For more information, see the following sources:

Adapted from American Psychological Association Services, Inc., "How to Do Group Therapy Using Telehealth," last modified April 10, 2020, https://www.apaservices.org/practice/legal/technology/group-therapy-telehealth-covid-19; Adapted from Health Resources & Services Administration, "Telehealth for Behavioral Health Care," last modified December 7, 2022, https://telehealth.hhs.gov/providers/best-practice-guides/telehealth-for-behavioral-health/group-teletherapy.

Defining Individual Goals

As a group instructor, working on the goals of each individual within the group can be challenging, especially if the members of your group are at different stages in the change continuum. For instance, one member may have the personal goal of being active at least five days a week for 30 to 45 minutes at a time. Another member might be satisfied by maintaining three days of activity steadily. For a third group member, trying one 10-minute brisk walk at some point during the course of the group will be a big achievement. One way to handle individual goal setting when members are at different stages of motivational readiness is to encourage members in stages 1 and 2 to set mainly process-oriented goals, while members in stages 3, 4, and 5 can be encouraged to set both process-oriented and physical activity behavior goals.

By process goals, we are referring to behaviors other than actual physical activity behavior that can help a person move along the stage continuum, such as reading about the benefits of physical activity, asking someone to be a walking partner, or finding a location to try a different type of physical activity (e.g., a large, empty parking lot to try in-line skating for the first time, parks with good hiking trails). Too often individuals and exercise promoters focus mainly on the physical activity behavior goals and place much less (or no) emphasis on process goals. As a result, people in the earlier stages drop out because they are not ready to set physical activity goals. Process goals also make good homework assignments to do between group sessions.

Physical activity goals can involve step counts and be related to the frequency, duration, intensity, and type of actual physical activity behaviors (e.g., taking three 15-minute brisk walks during a given week, maintaining 150 minutes of moderate-intensity physical activity per week for the next 2 months). In your role as group leader, you should help group members set both short- and long-term goals related to their physical activity behavior (see figure 7.6 in chapter 7 for a form that can be used for this purpose). You might define short-term goals as those that group members can accomplish in a week or two (e.g., increase daily step count by 10%), whereas long-term goals are those they can accomplish over months. Walking a predetermined distance (e.g., across the state), becoming fit enough to participate in a community walk, and achieving 10,000 steps per day are examples of long-term goals.

Regardless of the type of goal, encourage each group member to set SMART (specific, measurable, achievable, realistic, and time-bound) goals. By realistic, we mean that goals should be challenging yet attainable and thus enhance clients' confidence in their ability to be active. By measurable, we mean that goals should be articulated in such a way that the client and others can observe whether the outcome has been achieved. Clients will have difficulty determining whether they have achieved their goal of becoming healthier, but they can determine that they are able to walk farther or that their cholesterol level has dropped from 220 to 200. Working on goal setting in a group setting is a great way to teach this important skill. Group members can learn from each other how to articulate an activity goal in such a way that it can be observed and measured, and they can get ideas for their own goals as they listen to others.

Setting goals also provides a format that you can use to structure a standard group session. The following is a suggested format that you can use for each group session:

- Assess how group members did with their individual short-term goals over the past week and assess their progress toward their long-term goals.
- Present the topic for the current group session.
- Evaluate whether group members obtained the information they needed or hoped to receive, and if all the information you intended to convey for that session was covered.

- Have each member set a short-term physical activity or behavioral goal for the upcoming week.

To give you an idea of how a stage-based physical activity group might work, we discuss in the next section a program that provided stage-based behavioral skills training in a group format. A sample of the curriculum used in Project Active is in table 8.2.

Table 8.2 Lifestyle Curriculum and Targeted Behavioral and Cognitive Strategies

Week	Session title and group activity	Behavioral and cognitive processes
1	Getting to Know You—Monitoring sedentary pursuits, substituting active alternatives	Increasing knowledge, substituting alternatives
2	Understanding Barriers—Listing personal barriers and benefits, fitting short bouts of activity into daily life	Comprehending benefits, increasing healthy opportunities
3	Learning More—Setting goals, assessing enjoyable physical activities, demonstrating energy intensity	Increasing knowledge
4	Enlisting Aid—Identifying social support sources and types of support	Enlisting social support, committing yourself
5	Getting Confidence—Reflecting on overcoming barriers, problem-solving to overcome obstacles	Increasing self-efficacy
6	Scavenging for Physical Activity—Examining alternative, nontraditional ways to be physically active	Increasing healthy opportunities, substituting alternatives
7	Rewarding Yourself—Choosing appropriate rewards for reaching short- and long-term goals	Rewarding yourself, committing yourself
8	Time Management—Prioritizing daily activities to fit in physical activity	Decision-making, increasing healthy opportunities
9	Scouting Physical Activity in Your Community—Using maps and resource guides to find new activities	Increasing healthy opportunities, enlisting social support
10	Reviewing Goals—Using a step counter to monitor activity and set goals	Reminding yourself
11	Physical Activity Fair—Discussing and demonstrating favorite physical activities	Committing yourself, increasing self-efficacy
12	Cognitive Restructuring and Relapse Prevention—Learning how to change all-or-none thinking, planning for relapses	Substituting alternatives, comprehending benefits

LEARNING FROM A SAMPLE STAGE-BASED CURRICULUM

In Project Active (Dunn et al., 1997; Dunn et al., 1998), the lifestyle program was delivered as a group program in which about 15 participants at a time met with group facilitators who had training in psychology, health education, or exercise science for one hour, one night a week for the first four months, and then every other week for two more months. Meeting topics revolved around cognitive and behavioral skill building, developing self-efficacy for physical activity, solving problems, and focusing on the individual issues of both group members and facilitators. The goal was to help participants learn skills to enable them to integrate activities of at least moderate intensity into their daily lives. As self-efficacy and use of cognitive and behavioral skills increased, the program tapered to fewer group meetings (monthly and then bimonthly) throughout the remainder of the two-year program.

Similar theory-based group strategies have been successfully facilitated via social media and virtual platforms in recent studies. For example, researchers have used Facebook groups to host discussions on social cognitive theory constructs related to physical activity among cancer survivors (Pekmezi et al., 2022; ongoing) and African American women (Joseph et al., 2015). Joseph and colleagues (2015) scheduled weekly Facebook group posts every Wednesday (see examples below) that encouraged participants to share personal experiences with physical activity, give and receive social support for physical activity, and further target social cognitive theory constructs (table 8.3). Study staff did not participate in the Facebook group conversation, except to correct physical activity misinformation posted by a participant on one occasion. Findings from this African American female sample indicated that compared to a print-based intervention (PI), the Facebook interventions (FI) decreased sedentary time (FI = −74 min/wk vs. PI = +118 min/wk) and increased light intensity (FI = +95 min/wk vs. PI = +59 min/wk) and moderate-lifestyle intensity physical activity (FI = +27 min/wk vs. PI = −34 min/wk; all P's < .05).

Table 8.3 Stage-Based Curriculum

Week	Physical activity topic	Group discussion question	Social cognitive theory constructs targeted
1	Overview of the national physical activity recommendations, health benefits of physical activity, and physical activity statistics among African American women	What are your thoughts on the physical activity statistics among African American women? How can you incorporate more physical activity into your daily routine?	• Behavioral capability • Self-regulation
2	Developing a physical activity plan that works for you	What types of physical activity do you enjoy doing? What tips can you provide the group to help increase daily physical activity?	• Behavioral capability
3	Barriers to physical activity among African American women and strategies to overcome barriers	What are your specific barriers to physical activity, and what strategies will you use to help overcome them?	• Behavioral capability • Self-efficacy
4	Developing a social support network to promote physical activity	Who are potential sources of social support for physical activity?	• Social support
5	Strategies for incorporating short bouts of physical activity into your daily routine to achieve national physical activity recommendations	What strategies can you use each day to engage in more physical activity?	• Self-regulation
6	Testimonials from African American women on how they successfully incorporate physical activity into their daily lives	If you were to give a testimonial to other participants on how you maintain a physically active lifestyle, how would it sound?	• Outcome expectations
7	*Revisited:* National physical activity recommendations, barriers to physical activity among African American women, strategies to overcome barriers, and strategies to incorporate more physical activity into your life	How have you overcome the barriers to physical activity you had prior to starting the study?	• Behavioral capability • Self-regulation • Self-efficacy
8	Strategies for maintaining a physically active lifestyle after the intervention	How will you continue to be physically active?	• Outcome expectations

Rodney Joseph.

CASE EXAMPLE

CREATING CHANGE THROUGH GROUP COUNSELING

Sam, a 48-year-old engineer, was referred for group physical activity counseling because he had complained of having less energy and more trouble sleeping over the past year. Sam was pleased to join a virtual group because he knew he would not like attending face-to-face visits or the gym regularly. Yet he was skeptical about how much group support could help him given his busy work and personal schedule.

When Sam started, he was in stage 3 (doing some physical activity), had low self-efficacy for physical activity, identified several barriers that prevented him from being active (lack of time), and had made few steps toward becoming more active to date. However, Sam did play golf every Sunday, weather permitting, and carried his clubs when he played. In the first group discussion board, Sam reported that he saw no way to add physical activity during the week because of work demands. Moreover, he had no time to add activity on Saturdays because he blocked that out for family time. The group members encouraged Sam to think about adding physical activity in short bouts during his workday. Sam agreed to think about this and "liked" several discussion board posts in which group members described the strategies they used to fit exercise into their daily routine. Although Sam continued to assert that he could not change his weekday schedule much, he did begin to think that there might be a way for him to get in some activity regularly.

Sam noticed that he often got distracted and unproductive if he sat in front of his computer for more than an hour at a time. After a few weeks, Sam decided to try setting his phone's alarm to go off every hour. If he was sitting at his desk, he would get up and take a two-minute walk. During the next week, he found he could easily take three two-minute walks per day. Although he saw no increase in his productivity as a result, he also realized he did not lose any productivity despite these six minutes of walking per day.

With the support of two other group members with busy schedules, Sam first increased the number of times per day he took hourly walks, and then he increased the number of minutes of some walks. As a result, four months into the program, Sam was taking two 2-minute walks, two 5-minute walks, and two 10-minute walks on a typical weekday. He found that not only did he not lose any productivity, but he actually was more productive during the week because of these walking breaks. Moreover, he was now getting at least 30 minutes of moderate-intensity physical activity most days of the week and was still playing golf on Sunday. Best of all, his wife said he was less irritable with the kids and more engaged in family dinnertime conversation! Sam was now in stage 4 (doing enough physical activity), and he was optimistic that he could sustain this new habit.

Incorporated into the Project Active group meetings curriculum were the 10 processes of change, self-efficacy, and decision-making for physical activity (see chapters 2, 3, and 4), which are part of the stages of motivational readiness for change model (Prochaska & DiClemente, 1983) and social cognitive theory (Bandura, 1986, 1997) that can be applied to physical activity adoption and maintenance. These ideas were the basis of the strategies for building self-efficacy and cognitive and behavioral skills. Samples of activities from the six-month curriculum and the corresponding psychological processes are shown in table 8.2. The full curriculum is available in the book *Active Living Every Day* (Blair et al., 2021).

ASSESSING YOUR EFFECTIVENESS AS A LEADER

To determine whether you, as the group leader, achieved your objective for a session or topic, you can use group discussion, such as reviewing information provided in group meetings and how participants have applied various concepts and strategies. You might also consider obtaining more formal feedback by administering questionnaires to help you determine if they consider the information covered in group discussion useful. Here are some survey items you might consider having the participants fill out anonymously.

Participant satisfaction

Overall, I rate this session as

- Excellent
- Good
- Fair
- Poor

How useful was the information covered in today's group discussion?

- Very useful
- Somewhat useful
- Somewhat useless
- Completely useless

What did you like most about the session?
What did you like least about the session?
The group leader explained today's session content clearly and concisely.

- Strongly agree
- Agree
- Disagree
- Strongly disagree

What did the group leader do well today?
What could the group leader have done better today?
Overall, I rate the group leader's effectiveness as

- Excellent
- Good
- Fair
- Poor

You could also look for improvements in the content covered as a metric of success. If the session's topic was self-efficacy, you might want to have participants complete the confidence (self-efficacy) questionnaire found in appendix A at the beginning of the session so that they can identify areas in which they are more or less confident. Then, after spending the session discussing ways to stay active in challenging situations such as vacations and bad weather, you might have them fill out the questionnaire again to see whether there have been any improvements in self-efficacy. If there is no standardized measure available for the topic you covered, you can have participants answer a few questions about the content covered to see how well they learned the information.

You do not necessarily have to collect participants' responses to questionnaires or questions; this could just be a way for participants to reflect on their progress. Alternatively, this survey data could be used to provide specific feedback for participants to read and consider privately (strategies for increasing confidence in the areas in which they are struggling).

You may also want to encourage group members to track their progress and discuss challenges with the group. Some examples of useful content to include in a physical activity diary are provided in chapter 6 (see figures 6.1, 6.3, and 6.5).

Stage-Specific Suggestions for Group Activities

In this section we provide some strategies that you can incorporate into your own group curriculum. You can select among the options based on the stages of motivational readiness of your participants. If your group consists mainly of people who are in the same or similar stages of change, you might use the strategies described under the appropriate stage. If you find that your group has members in both the earliest stages (i.e., 1 or 2) and the later stages (i.e., 4 or 5), you might find it easier to break the group into smaller subgroups to adequately address the needs of each member. We would also encourage you to come up with your own ideas for group activities based on your setting and the needs of your clients.

Stage 1: Not Thinking About Change

You may find that some people in this earliest stage joined the group but are not currently interested in considering physical activity. Perhaps they joined to please someone else, such as a physician or family member. Or maybe they initially joined the group because they were in stage 2 or 3 but then regressed to an earlier stage during the course of the group. Let them know that they can still participate in meetings and chats even if they are not interested in starting physical activity right now, because they may get some ideas that will be helpful if they want to be active later. Some of the following strategies may encourage them to think about trying physical activity again, or perhaps for the first time.

What might you do to keep these people involved in your group?

- Determine their willingness to participate in discussions or do other behavioral assignments, such as looking up the benefits of physical activity.
- Lead a discussion about how people's sedentary behavior might affect those around them.
- Discuss another relevant health behavior (e.g., smoking cessation, healthy eating) and relate physical activity to this behavior.
- Discuss past attempts at becoming physically active. Is this related to why they are not interested in change now?
- Ask if you can check in with them every month or so to see where they are with physical activity.
- Foster social support from other group members for those who are still attending the group meetings even though they are not thinking about becoming physically active now.
- Ask them to list any barriers to physical activity.
- Administer the Physical Activity Readiness Questionnaire (figure 7.1) and address health events that might preclude physical activity.
- Lead a group discussion on barriers to physical activity.
- Consider addressing body image. Listen for any clues that suggest that some members are concerned about how they might look while engaged in physical activity.
- Ask them what they would need to consider doing physical activity.
- Present recommended levels of physical activity and the benefits that can be gained through accumulated moderate-intensity physical activities.
- List lifestyle activities that can help them achieve health benefits if performed at a moderate intensity (see chapter 6 for ideas). Notions such as "no pain, no gain" may be leading some to remain at this stage.
- Invite a guest speaker to discuss the benefits of physical activity.
- Consider some goals that might help these people move toward considering change.

- Ask these group members to think about a behavior, other than physical activity, that they were successful at changing and generate a list of strategies that were helpful in these past attempts.
- Ask group members to generate a list of common negative thoughts concerning physical activity and identify alternative positive thoughts they could use to replace them.

Stage 2: Thinking About Change

Group members in stage 2 are thinking about becoming more active and will probably find support from other group members helpful in their efforts to move toward actually trying this new behavior. Ideas from other group members who are participating in physical activity can help members in stage 2 to carefully plan their initial attempts at physical activity so that the experience is pleasant enough to try again. Here are some ideas for helping group members who are thinking about change.

What information might help these group members consider trying some physical activity?

- Present various types of social support (described in chapter 4). Have each participant identify areas in which social support would be helpful in getting started.
- Ask them to list barriers to physical activity.
- Use the IDEA approach described in chapter 7 to teach group members how to overcome perceived barriers. Have group members practice this problem-solving approach with each other or on their own (see figure 7.5).
- Lead a group discussion on priority setting and where beginning physical activity fits in their list of priorities.
- Ask participants to list activities that might help them get started.
- Set up teams to investigate various aspects of physical activity (e.g., benefits of cardiorespiratory activities, benefits of weight training, mental health benefits of physical activity, local places to go swing dancing).
- Through group discussion, develop strategies for obtaining social support and rewarding others who provide social support.
- Discuss activities that people in stage 2 might like to try or find enjoyable.
- Encourage group members to plan when, where, and with whom they might try some of these activities.
- Think of ways in which some light activities can be stepped up a notch into moderate-intensity activities (see chapter 6).
- For participants who are ready, set a date for trying a physical activity and post this information on social media, a bulletin board, and other visible locations to build commitment.
- Consider goals that might help these participants move toward change. Doing this in group discussions can be greatly beneficial because one

participant can learn from another. Stating goals and publicly committing to plans to meet said goals can enable group members to provide suggestions for helping others reach their goals.

- Ask group members to talk to someone they know who was successful at becoming physically active and get that person's advice. Have them share this advice with each other at the next meeting.
- Have each group member complete a personal time study to monitor the time spent sitting and the time spent engaging in some physical activity during two typical weekdays and a typical weekend day (see chapter 6). Brainstorm ideas for decreasing sedentary time and increasing time spent in physical activity.
- Plan a 10-minute walk either during group time or for participants to try on their own during the next week.

Stage 3: Doing Some Physical Activity

Participants in this stage are doing some physical activity but are not yet meeting national guidelines. Group discussion that provides these people with additional ideas and strategies for increasing their activity levels will be helpful, as will support from other group members. Be sure to encourage goal setting for both behavioral skills and actual physical activity behaviors. Here are some ideas for group members at this stage.

What are the remaining barriers?

- Choose an obstacle that is interfering with physical activity for one or several of the group members.
- Use the IDEA approach described in chapter 7 to develop potential solutions for overcoming this barrier.
- Practice with other obstacles.
- Work with group members on setting appropriate goals for gradually increasing their physical activity.
- Present various types of social support (described in chapter 4). Ask each participant to identify areas in which social support would be helpful in becoming more active. Through group discussion, develop strategies for obtaining social support and rewarding others who provide social support.
- Generate a list of rewards for achieving personal goals. Also, describe how one might use a point system to reward progress over time.
- Ask group participants to complete the processes of change questionnaire found in appendix A and get feedback from others on how they could implement additional change strategies.
- Have group members brainstorm ways to remind themselves to be more active.
- Ask group members to interview someone they know who was successful at becoming regularly active and get that person's advice. Have them share this advice with each other.

- Have some group members post short videos about the activities they like to do.
- Encourage short-term physical activity goals that are realistic and manageable. For example, people in stage 3 might consider increasing their current duration of physical activity per day by 5 or 10 minutes or their frequency of physical activity by one day.

Stage 4: Doing Enough Physical Activity

Even though group members in stage 4 are physically active at the recommended level, their challenge will be to maintain physical activity over time. They will still benefit from physical activity information and from setting both behavioral and physical activity goals. Here are some suggestions for helping regularly active group members stay active.

What information might help these participants continue physical activity until it is a habit?

- Encourage group members to share ideas on alternative activities to help prevent boredom.
- Lead a discussion on how others can unintentionally (or intentionally) sabotage their best efforts to stay active. How have others overcome this issue?
- Discuss how group members have encouraged others to be supportive.
- Invite a guest to talk about or demonstrate a new type of activity such as tai chi, yoga, or kickboxing.
- Post information on local hiking or biking trails.
- Discuss ways to monitor activity such as wearable devices (e.g., pedometers, wristbands), smart phone applications, heart rate monitors, and activity logs.
- Discuss the importance of rewarding oneself for accomplishing personal goals.
- Discuss common obstacles that can arise and get even the most dedicated exercisers off track (see chapter 7).
- Try a new activity as a group (e.g., ice skating at a nearby rink).
- Encourage group members to identify a role model who helps to motivate them.
- Have group members generate a personal list of rewards for physical activity.
- Ask group members to share what they have given up to become physically active or what they still find unpleasant about physical activity. Discuss ways to address these issues.
- Work on appropriate goal setting to maintain motivation over the long term.
- Start a discussion thread on what types of benefits participants believe they have already achieved. What benefits are they still working toward?

- Problem-solve as a team about any remaining obstacles some group members may still be experiencing.
- Have group members brainstorm ways they might post reminders in their environments to praise themselves for their success.

Stage 5: Making Physical Activity a Habit

Participants in stage 5 are quite knowledgeable about physical activity. However, group counseling can still be a valuable source of support and additional ideas. Goals can be to review what has helped them remain active, encourage them to think of new ways to keep activity enjoyable, and formulate a plan for any future setbacks. Here are some ideas for group activities relevant to those who have managed to stay active over time.

What kind of group activities might foster continued physical activity maintenance?

- Encourage group members to share ideas for a variety of fun activities to help prevent boredom.
- Post pictures and information on local hiking or biking trails.
- Discuss ways to track activity (see chapter 6).
- Discuss the importance of continuing to reward oneself for achieving personal goals. Have group members generate a personal list of rewards.
- Emphasize the importance of appropriate goal setting to maintain motivation over the long term.
- Spend time identifying possible setbacks and developing plans to prepare for and overcome them.
- Have participants try to think of alternative, nontraditional ways to be active.
- Encourage participants to become physical activity mentors to people they know who are less active.
- Discuss how members can change all-or-none thinking should they find themselves getting off track.

CONCLUSION

Physical activity group-based counseling can be a fun and effective way of sharing ideas and allowing your clients to support each other in their efforts to be more physically active. Two (or more) heads are better than one, especially with exercise. Group physical activity counseling is often provided in person but can be offered virtually (via social media, video conferencing, etc.). Your role as the group leader will vary (teacher, motivator, facilitator, analyzer, consultant), depending on the stages of motivational readiness of your group members. The goals that you set for your group and for each individual in the group will also differ according to participants' stages of motivational readiness (process-oriented vs. physical activity goals). Tips and best practices for promoting social support for physical activity, navigating virtual settings, and assessing your effectiveness as a group leader were provided. The Project Active curriculum helped illustrate the incorporation of the stages of change and the processes of change into group sessions and activities. Examples of how to conduct such theory-based physical activity counseling groups via social media were also provided. Finally, the chapter outlined appropriate group activities specific to each stage of motivational readiness for physical activity you might encounter as a group leader.

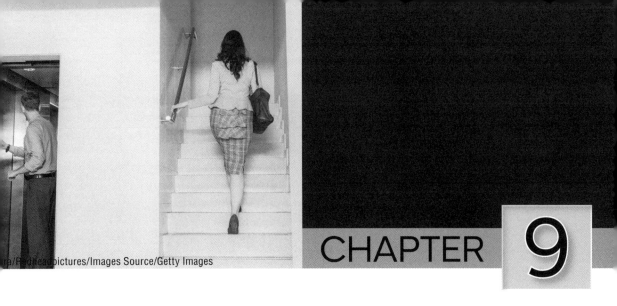

CHAPTER 9

Using the Stages Model in Worksite Programs

Office workers are sedentary for over 70 percent of their working hours, and half of all weekday sitting time is work related (Clemes et al., 2014; Kazi et al., 2014; Miller & Brown, 2004).

Thus, workplace physical activity programs offer great opportunities for helping many sedentary people become more active. While we use the terms *workplace* and *worksite* in this chapter, we would also like to acknowledge the growing trends in remote and hybrid work and address specific physical activity challenges your clients who work from home may face. Regardless of their employment setting, many people believe that the hours they spend working interfere with the time they have available for physical activity. This does not have to be the case. In fact, interventions conducted at worksites can be quite effective in increasing physical activity (Abdin et al., 2018; Buckingham et al., 2019; Burn et al., 2019; Jirathananuwat & Pongpirul, 2017; MacEwen et al., 2015; Muir et al., 2019; Shrestha et al., 2018).

> ### LEARNING HOW IT WORKS
> **Helping Clients Stay Active While Working Remotely**
>
> In today's economy, you can expect to encounter clients who work from an office, home, or both (hybrid). According to Census data, the number of people working from home tripled from 2019 to 2021, growing from 9 to 27.6 million people. While this was mostly due to the COVID-19 pandemic, many did not return to the office. Working from home has numerous perks for employers (e.g., more working hours from employees, increased productivity and profits; Osibanjo et al., 2022) and employees (e.g., short commute, relaxed dress code), but it can quickly lead to an inactive lifestyle. Your clients no longer need to walk to and from the office, conference room, and break room and can easily spend the whole day on the couch. Household tasks (e.g., laundry, dishes) can creep into time that was used for physical activity. While many of this chapter's worksite physical activity tips will translate, here are some special considerations for helping clients stay active while working from home. Encourage your clients to do the following:
>
> - Wear workout clothes. There is no need to wear a suit while working from home.
> - Keep sneakers and exercise equipment nearby. Be ready to do some physical activity during breaks.
> - Leave free weights, resistance bands, and other exercise equipment in plain sight as reminders.
> - Schedule exercise sessions. Put them in the daily planner.
> - Consider dedicating the time once spent commuting in the morning to working out.
> - Set a timer for a reminder to stand up and move for a few minutes every hour. It is easy to lose track of sitting time when working from home.
> - Work standing at the kitchen counter or a standing desk for a while each day.
> - Try taking at least one work call (non-video) while walking outside.
> - Start a virtual physical activity group with some like-minded coworkers. Just pick a time, connect via video call, and workout together from home.
>
> Adapted from Penn Medicine, "Staying Active While Working From Home," last modified March 19, 2020, https://www.pennmedicine.org/updates/blogs/heart-and-vascular-blog/2020/march/working-from-home.

Work environments can be arranged to provide opportunities for physical activity. Reminders to use the stairwell instead of the elevator can be posted, walking routes both inside the building and outside on the grounds can be marked and measured, and exercise equipment and facilities can even be provided. Furthermore, the workday actually provides hidden opportunities for activity so that employees can go home having already accumulated 30 minutes. Using coffee breaks to take 5- or 10-minute walks, holding one-on-one meetings while walking, and using the stairs instead of the elevator are examples of how this can be done. Using treadmill desks in workplaces produces improvements in several physiological outcomes (i.e., postprandial glucose, HDL cholesterol, and anthropometry; MacEwan et al., 2015). Standing desks and under-desk pedal exercisers are other strategies for making the workspace more conducive to movement.

The workplace can be an ideal place for disseminating physical activity–related information. Office settings typically have communication channels in place, such as email, websites, messaging applications, voice mail, newsletters, bulletin boards, and mailboxes, that can be useful for providing information about the benefits of physical activity or physical activity opportunities. Moreover, many workplaces offer built-in social support networks that you can use to spread your message and encourage employees in their efforts to be more active. Mobile health strategies (e.g., physical activity trackers, smartphone applications) can also serve as helpful prompts for worksite physical activity interventions (Buckingham et al., 2019).

Despite their value, worksite physical activity programs traditionally recruit only the employees who are already active to some degree (Marshall et al., 2004; Sharratt & Cox, 1988; Shephard, 1992). There is also a need for effective interventions for more sedentary employees. Worksite programs based on the stages of motivational readiness for change model are relevant and helpful even for those who are not interested in making behavior change in the foreseeable future. Such programs, which foster a positive attitude toward physical activity and create a social norm that supports good health and positive health habits, may move the least motivated people closer to adopting some physical activity or at least thinking about becoming more active soon. These employees may later decide to participate in activities either at home or at other facilities in the community. This chapter discusses general issues regarding the stage-matched approach for worksite programs and strategies that can be implemented in stage-matched workplace interventions.

BUILDING SUPPORT FOR YOUR PROGRAM

Before you begin developing and implementing your worksite program, you will need to consider the employer's commitment to your efforts. For example, if you want employees to participate in assessments of motivational readiness while at work, then managerial support for using work time for this purpose is clearly necessary. Selling your program to the employer by explaining the benefits of increasing the mental and physical well-being of the staff is well worth your time and effort.

> ### LEARNING HOW IT WORKS
> #### "Selling" Worksite Physical Activity to Management
>
> When leading a worksite physical activity program, it is important to emphasize how this will benefit employers, management, and other stakeholders. Their backing will be critical to program success in terms of securing the necessary time, resources, and support. Here are some key talking points that might help address employer and management priorities:
>
> - *Better work performance:* Physical activity improves creativity, memory, learning, and concentration. In fact, a U.K. study of nearly 200 white-collar employees found better performance, mood, time management, and job satisfaction on the days they exercised at work. The employees also reported not losing their temper, yelling, or slamming phones as much, which sounds particularly appealing to management and was probably related to stress management (Coulson et al., 2008).
> - *Stress management:* Stress can interfere with workers' ability to think clearly, focus, and make good decisions. Exercise at work can help employees manage stress through numerous mechanisms (e.g., reducing cortisol levels, releasing endorphins). Managers would probably rather not deal with stressed employees.
> - *Better health:* Employees who exercise regularly are generally healthier than those who are less active. Physical activity lowers the risk of heart disease, high blood pressure, diabetes, asthma, chronic pain, arthritis, and certain types of cancer. Physical activity also supports healthy weight maintenance and immune functioning. Thus, workplace physical activity programs can mean fewer sick days, medical appointments, and later retirement for employees, as well as substantial savings for employers (Kohl, 2019).

ASSESSING MOTIVATIONAL READINESS

To target your physical activity program at employees based on their stages of motivational readiness for change, you need a means of assessment that is quick and easy. You could administer questionnaire 2.1 in appendix A and use this information to gauge your approach and provide appropriate stage-matched physical activity messages. To provide more immediate feedback (and avoid excess paper waste), you could send the survey to employees via email or text message. If there are any concerns regarding literacy levels or visual impairments, automated telephone calls can be used to collect this data and provide appropriate physical activity counseling based on the responses, as in our past efforts (Brown et al., 2021).

Because people's stages of readiness for change fluctuate, you should assess employees' stages at several points in the program, depending on its length. Some programs have conducted stage assessments at the beginning, at one month, and at three months (Marcus et al., 1998); however, there is no strict rule for how often stage assessment should be done. How frequently you assess participants' behavior and physical activity intentions and what you use to assess their behavior depends on your program goals and ultimately the type of change you need to demonstrate to continue to receive funding or to attract new funding for your program.

CHOOSING YOUR TARGET AUDIENCE

One of your first decisions when designing a worksite program will be whether to recruit participants reactively (i.e., potential participants come to you) or proactively (i.e., you reach out to potential participants and offer your services).

If you decide to start with reactive recruitment strategies (i.e., intervening only with employees who have responded to your program advertisements rather than reaching out to all employees), you will need to have ideas for helping people at various stages of motivational readiness. However, if you proactively recruit participants, you can decide which stage you want your program to target and how you will reach people in that stage.

You may want your first program to focus on those in stage 3, who do some physical activity each week, and help them become regular exercisers. These people are an easy first target for your program because they are likely to be quite receptive to physical activity messages and events, and they have some ideas about how to get started. To reach them, you could sponsor a fun event, such as an "exercise journey," in which you pick a destination, such as a theme park, track the time or miles it would take to walk, jog, or swim there, and reward participants when they reach the destination. Such an event promotes the idea that physical activity is important and fun and encourages your target group members to monitor their progress and reward themselves for reaching a goal. If this event is successful, you can plan how to reach employees at other stages.

Although already active, employees in stage 4, doing enough physical activity, and stage 5, making it a habit, are often the people most interested in physical activity programs offered at work. Special events such as fun runs, fitness assessments, or rewards for physical activity participation can keep them motivated by making physical activity fun and different from their usual routine. Employees in these stages also are likely to be interested in tips for maintaining their activity during difficult times, such as bad weather or illness, and in information about unfamiliar exercise benefits, such as improved immune functioning. A short monthly newsletter or email message can provide these tips and information. The fact that these people are already active at the recommended level does not mean that they have little to gain from physical activity promotion. In fact, helping them vary their activities to prevent boredom and relapse is especially important because physical activity behavior is characterized by several starts and stops during a person's lifetime.

Employees in the earliest stages (i.e., stage 1, not thinking about change, and stage 2, thinking about change) are probably the ones that health promoters most want to reach. However, their lack of motivational readiness makes them the hardest to involve in worksite physical activity events. Your task is to increase these employees' awareness of the importance of physical activity, reinforce the notion that *anyone* can be physically active, and get them to think about how their current inactivity might affect them and others who are important to them. For this group, motivationally targeted messages that acknowledge their reluctance to become physically active are paramount. For example, ideas for overcoming common barriers may attract these people's attention because they believe that the reasons for being inactive outweigh those for being active. A heading such as "Not Ready to Be Physically Active?" communicates to employees at early stages that the information provided is relevant to them.

Messages aimed at people in the earlier stages and events for employees in the later stages communicate to all employees that physical activity is important to and valued by the employer. This can be crucial in moving people, even in the earliest stages, toward actually participating in some physical activity.

REACHING YOUR TARGET AUDIENCE

A common way to communicate physical activity messages in the workplace is to post them in highly visible places: websites, bulletin boards, break rooms, and doorways. Sending questions and receiving answers by email is another good option for many worksites. However, people who do not have a current interest in becoming more physically active may not pay much attention to these messages or may quickly dismiss them as irrelevant. Therefore, consider other communication channels that employees routinely use: social media, text messaging, and voicemails. Messages from the CEO, direct supervisors, employee health, managers, other employees, the human resources department, employee assistance programs, and union leaders may convince people in the early stages of motivational readiness to at least give physical activity another thought. Using several channels of communication also demonstrates to employees the organization's commitment to physical activity promotion.

DEVELOPING STAGE-MATCHED MATERIALS

In addition to information on the exercise facilities available or how to start an exercise program, be sure to also have available physical activity content geared toward people not thinking about activity and those thinking about it but not yet ready to start. This might include a podcast on the benefits of regular activity or suggestions for how to deal with common barriers that keep people from exercising. The early episodes should applaud the employee for taking the important first step of listening to information and learning about exercise. It is helpful to acknowledge in the title or the opening text that the employee may not be thinking of starting a physical activity program now but that the information might be useful if the person starts thinking more seriously about becoming physically active in the future. For example, we have used titles such as "What's in It for Me?" and "Do I Need This?" on content designed for people in stage 1. This helps people in the early stages perceive the messages as relevant to them, thereby increasing the likelihood that they will actually pay attention. Those in the later stages are seeking different information, such as how to prevent injury, how to add variety to their usual physical activity routines, or how to be active during vacations. Here are some suggested topics for stage-matched content:

Stage 1: Not Thinking About Change

- Health benefits of physical activity
- Overcoming common barriers

Stage 2: Thinking About Change

- Increasing lifestyle activity
- Considering benefits and barriers
- Setting short- and long-term goals

Stage 3: Doing Some Physical Activity

- Goal setting
- Developing a walking program
- Tips for enjoying physical activity
- Fitting more activity into a busy schedule

Stage 4: Meeting Physical Activity Guidelines

- Overcoming obstacles
- Preventing boredom
- Gaining social support
- Increasing your confidence in staying active

Stage 5: Making Physical Activity a Habit

- Avoiding injury
- Trying new activities
- Planning for difficult situations
- Rewarding yourself

FOCUSING ON MODERATE-INTENSITY ACTIVITY

Many people still adhere to the adage "no pain, no gain" with physical activity. This philosophy is particularly unappealing to those who are in the early stages of motivational readiness for physical activity. A worksite program based on the stages of change should promote activities that take little time or effort, consistent with the philosophy that any activity is better than none. Such activities include taking the stairs rather than the elevator, parking in the farthest parking space, or taking a walking break. Ask employees and managers to find opportunities for physical activity breaks throughout the workday to increase the effectiveness of your program.

Some businesses and employers might be reluctant to promote physical activity because they are concerned about liability issues should an employee become injured because of a program they have promoted. However, requiring that each employee consult with a physician before beginning a physical activity program puts up another barrier. You can address this concern by letting the employer know that moderate-intensity physical activity is low risk. Using the Physical Activity Readiness Questionnaire (see chapter 7) to identify any potential health concerns can allay employers' concerns about this issue.

PLANNING EVENTS

Action-oriented work events (e.g., virtual step contests, walkathons) and supportive policies and resources (e.g., exercise facilities, bicycle storage, shower and changing stations, flexible dress code) are a great place to start. However, a stage-matched workplace program should also include events that are more personal and skill building. An example of an activity targeted at employees in the early stages of motivational readiness could be brief emails with links to articles on the health benefits of physical activity. Encourage employees to share the physical activity articles or websites they found helpful so that you create a library of useful materials to distribute to other employees. Another idea is to ask employees to identify how they might benefit from becoming physically active and what barriers there are to being active. Provide aggregate feedback on the responses, along with problem-solving strategies. Start a work meeting by giving an active coworker or guest speaker a few minutes to describe the positive effects physical activity has had on their life. Provide employees with activity-related incentives, such as exercise bands, pedometers, and water bottles.

Employees in the early stages of motivational readiness may not be interested in becoming more physically active at present, but they might be interested in related issues, such as managing weight, stress, or time. Addressing these topics can help enhance their interest and confidence in physical activity; for example, you can encourage them to use their new time management skills to fit some activity into their schedule or persuade them that a little physical activity can be helpful in their efforts to manage their weight. Thus, programs and resources (e.g., via web-based platforms, smartphone applications, webinars) on these related mental and physical health topics can be a great use of your time and of management's financial resources.

ADDING INCENTIVES FOR PARTICIPATION

The idea of incentivizing participation comes from behavioral economics (discussed in earlier chapters), which assumes that people value the present more than the future. Thus, your client may skip physical activity today to return work emails because the immediate "costs" of physical activity (time spent) seem more pressing than the long-term health benefits. Financial incentives can help worksite programs overcome immediate opportunity costs and make physical activity more appealing to employees (Heise et al., 2021). Incentives for participation in workplace physical activity interventions, even self-funded commitment contracts (Royer et al., 2015), have been shown to increase programs' effectiveness (Dishman et al., 1998). Including several incentives for participation, especially in the beginning, helps employees commit to the program. Financial incentives include additional payments or reimbursements for participation. An employer might collaborate with a local exercise facility to offer a one-month membership to employees who sign up for the program. Prizes such as T-shirts, either for participation, physical activity tracking, syncing wearable devices, or meeting physical activity goals, have also been used. Workplace announcements (e.g., social media and newsletter spotlights) can be a great way to recognize participant efforts and help create social norms for physical activity. Release time from work to participate in physical activity has also been used as an incentive to get employees to participate, although this requires management's support. A systematic review of incentives for physical activity emphasized that rewards (for physical activity behavior vs. attendance) are more effective in influencing physical activity outcomes than unconditional incentives (e.g., free gym membership; Jeroen et al., 2017), which has important implications for best practices for incentivizing physical activity in a worksite setting.

Stage-Specific Strategies for Worksite Programs

Once you have evaluated employee interest and managerial support for your worksite physical activity promotion program, the funds you have available, and the means you are going to use to deliver the program, it is time to put it together. We hope that the following list of stage-specific workplace program strategies will help you generate some ideas for developing a program that will meet the needs of the employees with whom you are working.

Stage 1: Not Thinking About Change

For sedentary employees who are not thinking about physical activity behavior change, an appropriate objective for your program might be to increase their awareness of the benefits of physical activity and the level of activity necessary to obtain these benefits. Here are some strategies for increasing awareness and encouraging these employees to begin to think about the role physical activity could play in their lives.

What are some ways to promote physical activity awareness?

- Kick off your program with a special event, such as a guest speaker or by giving T-shirts to every employee.
- Place informational displays in prominent places such as the home page of the company website, the front entrance of the building, in reception areas, by the elevator or stairwell, on bulletin boards, at coffee or snack machines, or in the restrooms. Information can be sent via email and posted on social media.
- Offer an incentive to employees who read or find information on physical activity.
- Distribute information targeted toward people who are currently not thinking about becoming more physically active.
- Host a health fair that includes fitness testing, blood pressure screening, or body fat assessment. Relate how these are affected by physical activity.

What information might get employees to consider physical activity?

- Give a presentation to correct common misconceptions (e.g., you must exercise vigorously to gain health benefits).
- Present national physical activity guidelines and the benefits that can be gained through accumulated moderate-intensity physical activities.
- List lifestyle activities that can help a person achieve health benefits if performed at a moderate intensity (see chapter 6). Notions such as "no pain, no gain" may be leading some to remain at this stage.

What are some strategies for making physical activity personally relevant to these employees?

- Offer free physical fitness assessments.
- Do a barriers assessment related to either home or worksite physical activity and provide suggestions for overcoming barriers.
- Have employees identify how they might benefit from becoming physically active.
- Personalize your message to help employees see how it relates to their lives.
- Determine what the employees prioritize and tailor your activities to those goals (e.g., weight loss, mental health benefits).

What type of special event is particularly relevant for these employees?

- Hold a Top 10 Benefits T-Shirt Contest.
- Ask employees to submit the best benefits of exercising.
- Request two benefits—one that is legitimate and another that is funny.
- Have your employee wellness committee or other staff judge the benefits.
- Share highlights from the entries on social media.
- Order T-shirts printed with the top 10 benefits and offer them to all employees who participated.

Stage 2: Thinking About Change

For employees in stage 2, one of your objectives might be to increase awareness of the benefits of physical activity and its acceptance in the work community. A second objective would be to move these employees closer to actually trying the behavior. Here are some ideas for achieving these objectives.

What are some ways to promote physical activity awareness?

- Distribute information targeted toward people who are thinking about becoming more physically active.
- Establish an online library with educational materials on physical activity.
- Take advantage of New Year's resolutions in January or other dates to post information or hold an event.
- Kick off your program with a special event, such as a guest speaker or by giving T-shirts to every employee.
- Place informational displays in prominent places such as at the company website home page, front entrance, in reception areas, by the elevator or stairwell, on bulletin boards, at coffee or snack machines, or in the restrooms, or send information by email.
- Offer an incentive to employees who read or find information on physical activity.

What information might get employees to consider physical activity?

- Conduct a health fair that offers free physical fitness assessments. Offer virtual physical function assessments for those who work remotely (see Hoenemeyer et al., 2022, for more details).
- Gather and distribute a list of community and online resources for physical activity.
- Do a barriers assessment related to either home or worksite physical activity and provide suggestions for overcoming barriers.
- Hold a webinar on developing an activity plan (what, where, when, and with whom).

What strategies might prompt these employees to try some physical activity?

- Provide employees with the opportunity to take a 10-minute walking break during the workday. End regular meetings and conference calls 10 minutes early to allow time for physical activity.
- Post cues by the elevator to take the stairs instead.
- Have employees set a "start date," during which they will complete the goal of 10 minutes of physical activity. Follow up to see how the employees did.
- Give the message that "some activity is better than nothing."

What is an example of a special event that would be appropriate for employees in this stage?

- Host an event called Take a Walk in My Shoes.
- Plan a walking route that covers an appropriate distance (it can be a local walking path or a shopping mall).
- Select landmarks (stores, playgrounds) at intervals as "checkpoints" and note distinctive landmark features (interesting window displays and playground equipment).
- Create a scavenger hunt with a series of questions about the landmarks that participants must answer during the walk.
- Keep in mind that many of the participants will be sedentary, so be conservative with the distance you expect them to travel.
- Encourage participants to walk the route in pairs or participate virtually (by walking the designated distances on a treadmill or in their own neighborhood). Arrange incentives.

Stage 3: Doing Some Physical Activity

Employees in stage 3 are likely to be receptive to physical activity promotion in the workplace, given that they are doing some activity but not enough to meet national guidelines. Therefore, your program objective for this group is to encourage them to increase the amount of physical activity they do each week, perhaps by getting more physical activity in during work hours. To communicate with these employees about your program, you can use various communication channels available at the worksite. Here are some ideas to target these employees.

What channels might you use to get your message to these employees?

- Host a webinar on making time for physical activity or strategies for building in activity routinely throughout the day.
- Start an email program that offers a tip of the day and encourages employees to track their steps via wearable devices or logs. Provide encouragement and support through brief emailed feedback.

- Post energy expenditure charts on the company website and in physical meeting spots.
- Distribute brochures targeted toward people who are thinking about becoming more physically active. Provide digital copies via email and place hard copies in worksite common areas.

What strategies might help these employees increase their physical activity?

- Encourage these employees to keep track of how much activity they are doing each week.
- Create a point system for making progress toward a physically active lifestyle. Make points redeemable for meaningful rewards, such as donated gifts from local sponsors.
- Post cues by the elevator to take the stairs instead.
- Help to create informal physical activity support networks among the employees (e.g., walk meetups).
- Provide exercise prescriptions appropriate to employees' levels of fitness.
- Offer resources such as under-desk pedal bike exercisers, free weights, and standing or walking desks.
- Have employees monitor the minutes they spend sitting and being active during the day. Encourage employees to replace sitting time with activity time (see chapter 6).
- Encourage employees to hold one-on-one meetings while walking.
- Suggest that employees set their computers to beep once an hour as a reminder to take a two-minute walk.
- Encourage employees to set a realistic goal for increasing the amount of activity they are doing.
- Provide opportunities for employees to practice new physical activity skills in a safe, nonjudgmental environment.

What is an example of a special event that would be appropriate for employees in this stage?

- Plan an event called Conquering Mount Everest.
- To prepare for this journey, a few calculations are necessary.
- The total height of Mount Everest is 29,028 feet (8,848 m).
- The distance between floors in most office buildings is 13 feet (4 m).
- One way to structure this journey is to have participants climb 130 feet (40 m) per day (10 floors), five days per week.
- "Trek teams" with four members each would need approximately 11 weeks to complete the event.
- Designate one person as the "trail guide" to serve as team organizer and leader.

- Team members report their climbing success each week to the sherpa, who totals it and reports it to you. Encourage your employees to add stair climbing to their daily routines rather than trying to do a week's worth of climbing in one day.

Stage 4: Meeting Physical Activity Guidelines

Employees in stage 4 have recently become active at the level recommended by national guidelines. Your program objective for this group will be to promote continued participation in activity for the long term. To accomplish this, you can use some of the following strategies.

What channels might you use to get your message to these employees?

- Distribute information targeted toward people who are regularly physically active but only recently so.
- Use video conferencing calls and social media threads for physical activity problem-solving.
- Conduct a workshop or webinar on preventing boredom with physical activity.
- Start an email-based program that offers a tip of the day and encourages employees to track and email reports of their physical activity. Provide encouragement and support through brief emailed feedback.

What strategies might help these employees keep up their physical activity?

- Teach skills in alternative activities (e.g., in-line skating, tennis, kickboxing, martial arts–based workouts). Provide access to relevant online instructional videos.
- Encourage employees to create a plan for maintaining or resuming physical activity when work or life is especially hectic.
- Sponsor an event that includes family and friends. Provide wearable devices and exercise equipment for family and friends.
- Post mile markers on worksite grounds or measure the distance of inside routes.
- Negotiate deals for employees to use local exercise facilities.
- Give employees points for time spent being physically active each week and make points redeemable for small gift items, such as exercise clothing or passes to local exercise facilities.

What further activities would be appropriate for employees in this stage?

- Encourage physical activity social support. Use surveys, focus groups, and discussion boards to facilitate physical activity partnerships and establish what these employees need. Create an employee physical activity email list and send them supportive messages.

- Publicly announce your physical activity intervention efforts and establish an initial web meeting time, date, and place. Arrange for a content expert to be available at the initial meeting (and at future meetings on an as-needed basis). At the initial meeting, introduce your expert, determine the goals of the group, and share ideas for the group.
- Identify potential group leaders who can assist in communications and logistics. Establish a proposed meeting schedule and use your connections to set recurring video conferencing links, reserve rooms, and obtain management permission if needed.
- Attend occasional web meetings yourself to keep in touch with employees' activities and status.

Stage 5: Making Physical Activity a Habit

Employees in stage 5 are familiar with physical activity because they have been regularly active for at least six months. Your program objective will be to help them stay active by anticipating lapses, planning for situations that jeopardize their activity, and keeping them motivated over the long term. Here are some suggestions for achieving these goals.

What strategies might help these employees prevent setbacks in their physical activity?

- Distribute information targeted toward people who are active and have been so for at least six months.
- Sponsor a charity walk or run.
- Give away step counters and other wearable devices. Provide self-monitoring booklets or magnets with a self-monitoring form to encourage continued goal setting (see chapter 6). Offer tech support to set up related equipment and smart phone applications.
- Ask these employees to sponsor a friend, family member, or coworker who is trying to get started with physical activity.
- Give a webinar on injury prevention.
- Teach skills in alternative activities to prevent boredom.

What is an example of a special event that would be appropriate for employees in this stage?

- Organize a five-kilometer fun walk or run or a company field day. Consider including family members for team events (e.g., a caregiver and child relay race).
- Begin a walking or running program with a destination-based or distance goal (e.g., a 30-mile/month [48.3 km] challenge).
- Host a webinar on performing physical activity in inclement weather featuring tips on training methods and specialized clothing.

- Organize a series of online events featuring indoor physical activity options (e.g., walking on indoor tracks or treadmills) as alternatives to outdoor walking or running during inclement weather.
- Promote active participation in your walking club, especially for new members.
- Develop a list of locations, such as local colleges and community sport facilities, that are suitable for indoor physical activity during inclement weather. If possible, provide maps of the locations.

CONCLUSION

Because many Americans still work outside the home, worksite physical activity programs have the potential to reach many people and can capitalize on built-in communication, infrastructure, and support systems. We discussed worksite physical activity features that will likely appeal to management and employers because securing their buy-in early can be critical to program success. Recent trends in working from home and on hybrid schedules were described, along with challenges to staying active in these situations. It has never been easier to spend the entire day on the couch. Thus, we discuss how to help clients working from home find opportunities to move. Workplace physical activity programs primarily attract only those employees most motivated to be physically active. However, a stage-matched approach, as described in this chapter, can appeal to and retain greater numbers of employees than traditional programs can. We hope that this chapter has provided some useful ideas for developing and implementing a physical activity program to meet the needs of all employees, regardless of their motivational stage of change and workplace setting. Moreover, we have described how technology (e.g., standing desks and sitting time alerts on wristbands) can be used to help support employees when working in the office or at home.

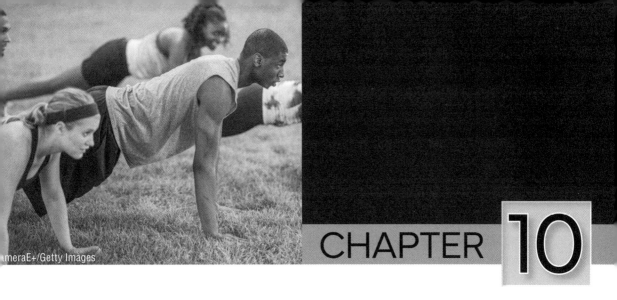

CHAPTER 10

Using the Stages Model in Community Programs

The first step to designing and implementing a community-based physical activity program is often defining the community. These days, community is not limited to geography and can refer to many things (e.g., virtual communities, such as Facebook groups). Developing a program to meet the needs of an entire community can be a daunting task. The people within any given community are sure to differ substantially, so whom should you target? What type of program can help these people the most? Such a large-scale project may also be expensive. However, community programs have the potential to reach a great number of under-active people through various channels, such as the mass media, print materials, and community leaders, and through organized events such as fun runs and health fairs. You can also reach a larger number of people in the community at a low cost per person by taking advantage of technologies such as the telephone, interactive computer systems, and the Internet (Larsen et al., 2017; Marcus, Owen, et al., 1998; Marcus, Lewis, et al., 2007; Marcus, Napolitano, et al., 2007 Marshall et al., 2004).

Community campaigns to improve cardiovascular health that have included physical activity have been around for decades. Programs such as the Stanford Five-City Project (Young et al., 1996) and the Minnesota Heart Health Program (Luepker et al., 1994) have targeted several cardiovascular risk factors, including high blood pressure, poor diet, and tobacco use, while promoting physical activity. In the past, community-based projects tended to use a one-size-fits-all approach, in which a general message promoting physical activity was given to all people, regardless of their level of motivational readiness for beginning physical activity. Although programs such as these helped increase awareness of the benefits of physical activity, they were less effective at increasing physical activity behavior (Marcus, Owen, et al., 1998).

We have since learned that it is important to divide the population into subgroups (i.e., target audiences) and customize programs for each of these segments to better meet the needs of people within a community and to have better recruitment and retention in programs. Studies that have divided populations by motivational stage of readiness and then delivered stage-targeted messages have proven to be more successful than traditional approaches for getting people to change their behavior (Golsteijn et al., 2018; Marcus, Bock, et al., 1998; Marcus, Emmons et al., 1998; Short et al., 2015; Will et al., 2004). Chapter 5 provides a more detailed description of some of these programs, such as Jump Start, Project STRIDE, and Step Into Motion.

In this chapter we discuss how you can use the stages of motivational readiness to design a physical activity program for the people in your community and strategies that might be effective for these people. You can also refer to "Strategies to Prevent Obesity and Other Chronic Diseases: The CDC Guide to Strategies to Increase Physical Activity in the Community" (Centers for Disease Control [CDC], 2011) for more information on designing and implementing community programs. To begin, we discuss reasons to use the stages of motivational readiness to build your program.

ASSESSING THE COMMUNITY'S READINESS FOR CHANGE

Traditionally, the stages of motivational readiness for change model is used to describe behavior change at the individual level (Glanz et al., 2015). However, some have also applied it to entire communities to describe how ready a given community is to make physical activity a priority for its residents (Abrams, 1991; Kehl et al., 2021; McLeroy et al., 1988; USDHHS et al., 1999). Researchers and health promoters alike have noted that environmental factors are important considerations for individual behavior change (Brown et al., 2023; Heath et al., 2006; Humpel et al., 2002; Kahn et al., 2002). For example, sidewalks and bike and walking paths enhance the likelihood of individual behavior change. Institutional factors also affect individual change, such as an employer who does not give employees release time for physical activity. The stages of physical activity readiness at a community level are also influenced by societal factors, such as support from community officials. As illustrated in figure 10.1, environmental, social, and institutional factors influence each other and are all important considerations in a community's readiness for change.

Here are other specific examples of how the stages of change can be interpreted at a community level:

- A worksite that is considering a change in employee health benefits to include physical activity incentives might be in stage 2, thinking about change.

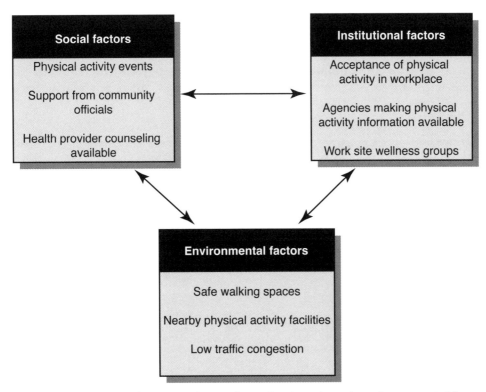

Figure 10.1 The influence of social, institutional, and environmental factors on community readiness for change.

- A worksite whose administration is already taking the appropriate steps to institutionalize a cost-effective physical activity program might be in stage 5, making activity a habit.
- A school district that is piloting a model physical activity program in one of its schools may be in stage 3, doing some physical activity, before adopting the program district wide.
- A community in the construction phase of converting old railroad lines into pedestrian and bicycle pathways has demonstrated that the community is in stage 4, or the action phase.

Determining the stage of motivational readiness of a community helps you learn the barriers to change at the community level (e.g., unsafe neighborhoods for walking, few activity-related events, lack of support from community officials) and the potential community supports for physical activity (e.g., health care providers willing to counsel their patients on physical activity, worksite wellness groups) already in place. The community's motivational readiness for physical activity promotion can be determined in various ways. You might examine the community's physical environment, or you might interview several community members of different ages, race/ethnicities, and so forth, to see whether they believe community support is in place for them to become or stay physically active (e.g., safe walking areas, acceptance of physical activity in the workplace, nearby community exercise facilities). You should also determine the community's commitment to physical activity–related goals or practices. For example, are agencies willing to make physical activity information available? Are activity-related events taking place?

LEARNING HOW IT WORKS
Assessing Physical Environment in the Community

How do you assess environmental support for physical activity in a community? You can use surveys, geographic information system data, or even conduct observations or audits to gain more information. The Neighborhood Environment Walkability Scale is a questionnaire commonly used in our (and other research teams') past studies (Almeida et al., 2021; Saelens et al., 2003). While this instrument includes 66 questions on residential density, land use mix, land use mix access, street connectivity, infrastructure for walking and cycling, aesthetics, traffic safety and hazards, and safety from crime, an abbreviated form is also available (Cerin et al., 2006). You can find both versions at www.drjimsallis.com. Environmental factors related to physical activity have also been measured with the Environmental Access Scale (Sallis et al., 1997). In past studies using this measure, we found improvements in perceptions on the availability of physical activity equipment and supplies in response to physical activity interventions (Pekmezi et al., 2009; Ries et al., 2009), which suggests that clients become increasingly aware of existing physical activity resources in the process of advancing through the stages of change and becoming more active.

We have also collected observational data on the physical activity environment in six underserved rural Alabama communities for the DIAL study (Brown et al., 2023). We used the Rural Active Living Assessment, which includes three components: the Town-Wide Assessment (TWA), the Program and Policy Assessment (PPA), and the Street Segment Assessment (SSA; Yousefian et al., 2010). The TWA has 18 town demographics and characteristic items (e.g., county population, town topography, and location of schools) and 15 recreational amenity questions (e.g., hiking, biking, and walking trails, parks, playgrounds, and recreational centers). The PPA consists of 11 questions evaluating the presence or absence of town and school programs (e.g., local public transportation, sponsored physical activity initiatives for students) and policies (e.g., requirement of bikeways or pedestrian walkways in new public infrastructure projects, public recreation department that offers physical activity programs) that could contribute to active living within the community. The SSA is a 25-item observational audit of individual street segments within the towns. This component characterizes walkability (e.g., sidewalks, safety features, and road and traffic characteristics), land use (e.g., residential, commercial, industrial, public, and civic), and aesthetics. See *Rural Active Living Assessment Tools: Codebook & Scoring* handbook (Hartley et al., 2009) for more details.

Overall, few town-wide amenities (TWA mean score = 49.67/100) or programs and policies for physical activity (PPA mean score = 24.67/100) were found in these rural communities. A total of 96 street segments were audited across the six counties (i.e., 16 segments across 18 towns) for the SSA. Few street segments boasted sidewalks (32%), shoulders in good condition (28%), or safety features, such as crossing signals (2%), children at play signs (6%), yellow school flashing lights (2%), and speed bumps (3%; Brown et al., 2023). Such data can provide important insights on existing physical activity–related resources and amenities, community programs, and policies. You can use these instruments to identify physical activity opportunities and environmental barriers that should be highlighted or addressed to help increase community physical activity.

Your stage assessment should include the community's status on physical activity–promoting actions, its intention to move toward them, and the steps it has taken or the plan it has in place for implementing them. You will also need to assess the community's ability to achieve specific behavioral goals related to physical activity. Such behavioral goals might include taking action in the following areas:

• *Social networks.* Develop community walking groups. Foster collaboration among local health agencies. Encourage partnerships between businesses and exercise facilities. Develop a hotline, email list, and social media campaign to offer ideas, information, and encouragement to members of the community.

• *Environment.* Raise funds for more biking and walking paths. Build housing developments near exercise facilities. Promote public transportation. Install better lighting for sidewalks.

• *Community norms.* Encourage biking with helmets as a way to travel to work. Publicize the need for childcare in fitness facilities. Start a walking school bus to encourage active transport to school. Have community leaders deliver physical activity messages.

• *Policies and legislation.* Lobby for tax cuts for worksites that promote physical activity for their employees. Pass zoning laws for green space. Require the inclusion of bikeways or pedestrian walkways in new public infrastructure projects. Advocate for school policies that allow public access to school recreation facilities after school hours.

Once you have determined the community's stage of motivational readiness for various program ideas that you have in mind, you can begin to think about how to meet the needs of individuals within the community.

REACHING INDIVIDUALS WITHIN A COMMUNITY

A goal of influencing everyone in a given community is unrealistic. Programs that try to do so end up serving no one very well. As mentioned earlier, general programs do not account for individual differences that affect physical activity adoption. A more appropriate goal for a community physical activity program is to reach a majority of people within the community.

To make a program work for a large number of people, you must assess the needs of the people you are trying to reach. You can determine the stages of most people in the community, or you can choose a target audience and then determine the stages of the people within it. Before designing your program, find out what the people in your target audience think about physical activity, why they might want to become more active, what has been holding them back, where they go to get their information, and possible sources of support. You can then customize your message to meet their needs.

This approach of designing your program around the needs and beliefs of your target audience derives from social marketing (Kotler & Zaltman, 1971). *Social marketing* is the use of business and marketing principles and strategies to influence behavior "for good" (i.e., to benefit the community and public health) and starts with listening to what consumers believe is best for them and formulating solutions to suit consumers' perceptions rather than trying to tell them what is best for them. Focus groups and interviews with the target audience can be conducted to solicit these consumer perceptions and further define the marketing mix for the campaign. The four *P*'s of the marketing mix include the product (physical activity), price (physical activity costs and barriers), place (where physical activity occurs), and promotion (messages and activities encouraging physical activity). Consider assessing the following when "marketing" physical activity programs for a community:

- the barriers versus benefits of the target behavior (e.g., lack of time for physical activity vs. potential chronic disease prevention);
- the barriers versus benefits of the competing behavior (e.g., watching TV is not great for health but enjoyable in the short term);
- the priorities and values of the community (e.g., health, happiness);
- how to make choosing the target behavior (i.e., being physically active) easier, more enjoyable, and popular (e.g., involve music, family, and friends);
- how, where, and when the target behavior occurs (e.g., at the park, on the weekends);
- who influences (i.e., creates opportunities for) the target behavior of the audience (e.g., parks and recreation departments, city administrators); and
- how the audience gets its information about the target behavior (e.g., signs, websites).

CASE EXAMPLE

CREATING CHANGE WITHIN THE COMMUNITY

Past research has shown that social marketing has been used with success to promote physical activity in different communities and populations (Kubacki et al., 2017; Xia et al., 2016), including older adults (Goethels et al., 2020). For example, the CDC employed social marketing principles in their Active People, Healthy Nation campaign and their I Choose campaign, with the goals of challenging social norms regarding physical activity and raising awareness of community resources and supports among the target audience (racial and ethnic minority adults and parents; Fulton et al., 2018). The resulting social media advertisements featured families (African American and Hispanic, in particular) engaging in free, low-cost physical activity in their communities (e.g., walking on sidewalks, playing soccer or football at the park). Analyses of social media metrics indicated that some messages ("I choose to play") caught more attention than others ("I choose to walk"). Targeting ads based on demographics and household income, among other metrics (e.g., zip code), helped improve reach and get more views compared to past efforts. Most social media views came from mobile users, which has implications for future campaigns (e.g., mobile-friendly websites).

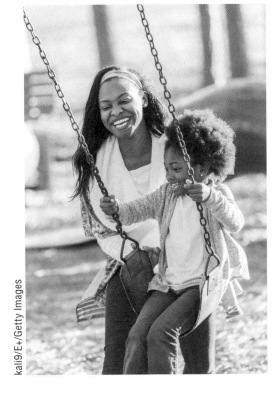
kali9/E+/Getty Images

Earlier CDC projects used similar social marketing techniques in different groups. For example, the VERB: It's What You Do! campaign for tweens focused on promoting physical activity as cool and fun (Huhman et al., 2017). The WISEWOMAN project (well-integrated screening and evaluation for women across the nation) demonstrated that social marketing approaches can yield positive results in middle-aged, financially disadvantaged women (Will et al., 2004), especially if the interventions are culturally and age appropriate, provide repeated exposure to physical activity opportunities, and increase social support (Stoddard et al., 2004).

DEVELOPING STAGE-MATCHED MESSAGES

Targeting and tailoring are two social marketing strategies that can be very useful for communicating physical activity messages (figure 10.2). Targeting a program involves defining groups within the population along some characteristic, such as stage of motivational readiness, and then delivering a program suited to this characteristic. A targeted approach assumes that the members of a defined group are similar enough for one message to effectively communicate to all members of the group. Targeting by stage of motivational readiness and then delivering stage-matched printed materials about physical activity have been shown to effectively increase physical activity behavior (Marcus et al., 1992; Marcus, Emmons, et al., 1998). Chapter 5 provides more detailed descriptions of these programs, such as Imagine Action and Jump Start: A Community-Based Study.

More recently, our intervention approaches have involved both *targeting* the general information needs and preferences of a group (e.g., in the preparation stage) and *tailoring* to individuals' concerns (Marcus et al., 2000, 2007, 2013, 2022; Marcus, Dunsiger, et al., 2015). Such approaches have outperformed more generic messages in achieving behavior change in numerous past studies (Noar et al., 2007). Tailored messages are more likely to be read, understood,

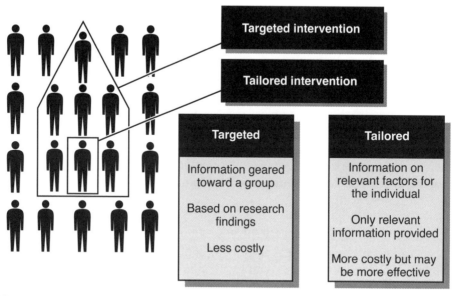

Figure 10.2 Targeted versus tailored approaches to physical activity promotion.

recalled, and considered credible (Kreuter, Farrell, et al., 2000; Kreuter & Holt, 2001; Noar et al., 2007; Rimer et al., 1994; Schmid et al., 2008), which might explain the appeal and persuasiveness of such communications.

Although providing individually tailored, stage-matched messages about physical activity sounds ideal, doing so is more expensive and labor intensive than delivering a single targeted message. You need to weigh the costs and benefits when deciding between a targeted and tailored approach (figure 10.3). In some cases, technologies such as computers and the Internet can be cost effective in individually tailoring physical activity messages. Moreover, technologies such as these allow us to move beyond reliance on face-to-face counseling to affordable, automated, individually tailored counseling (see chapter 5 for a description of programs that used computer-generated tailored messages, such as Jump Start: A Community-Based Study [Marcus, Bock, et al., 1998] and Project STRIDE [Marcus, Napolitano, et al., 2007]).

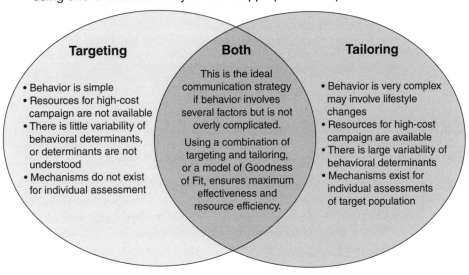

Figure 10.3 Factors to consider when deciding whether to use targeting, tailoring, or both.

Reprinted by permission from K.L. Schmid, S.E. Rivers, A.E. Latimer, and P. Salovey, "Targeting or Tailoring? Maximizing Resources to Create Effective Health Communications," *Marketing Health Services* 28, no. 1 (2008): 32-37, permission conveyed through Copyright Clearance Center, Inc.

> ### LEARNING HOW IT WORKS
> #### Tips on Tailoring
>
> How does one tailor a physical activity program? Which variables should be selected for tailoring? Tailoring can be accomplished by asking clients questions about their current level of physical activity self-efficacy, outcome expectations, and use of cognitive and behavioral strategies. This data can then be used to provide personalized physical activity advice via face-to-face counseling, mail, email, phone calls, websites, and text messages. For example, in our past studies, we targeted our messages to the general physical activity barriers of the population (e.g., underactive Spanish speaking Latinas), based on formative research, and tailored the advice to the specific information needs and concerns of the individual client, using theory as a guide for selecting the specific tailoring variables.
>
> Researchers have examined the added benefit of tailoring to client characteristics beyond the stage of change. For example, participants' gender and personality may influence how motivating they find certain advice. In one study (de Vries et al., 2017), certain personality characteristics (high openness) were associated with rating text messages on some processes of change (consciousness-raising and counterconditioning) as more motivating than others (on environmental revaluation). There were also differences by gender, with men rating text messages on consciousness-raising, dramatic relief, environmental reevaluation, and self-reevaluation as more motivating than women. Thus, when choosing motivational messages for physical activity, it may be important to consider individual factors such as gender and personality for optimal results.

USING A REMOTE APPROACH TO REACH YOUR TARGET AUDIENCE

Reviews of published physical activity studies reveal that community-based interventions delivered remotely (e.g., via print mailings, telephone, Internet) can be as effective as programs delivered face to face (Dishman & Buckworth, 1996; Joseph et al., 2014; Romeo et al., 2019; William et al., 2020). Remote interventions allow people more flexibility and choice in how they implement their physical activity programs, whereas face-to-face programs usually entail some type of physical activity done in the counselor's presence. Moreover, most households can be conveniently reached at a lower cost by mail, telephone, or the Internet.

Print

Print-based, stage-targeted physical activity programs delivered to sedentary adults by mail have been found to help them become more active (e.g., Cardinal & Sachs, 1996; Marcus et al., 1992), as have print-based, tailored, self-help physical activity programs (Marcus, Bock, et al., 1998). Participants can be mailed the stages of change questionnaire (questionnaire 2.1 in appendix A) along with other relevant measures, such as the processes of change, self-efficacy, and decisional balance questionnaires (questionnaires 4.1, 4.2, and 4.4 in appendix A). They can then receive personally relevant printed materials within a day or two of mailing their questionnaires. While these findings are from mostly White samples, such strategies have also been shown to be effective in promoting physical activity within underserved, at-risk populations (underactive African American and Latina women; Marcus et al., 2013; 2022; Marcus, Dunsiger et al., 2015; Pekmezi et al., 2009; 2017;2020).

Telephone

The telephone is another avenue for reaching large numbers of people within a community, given that most Americans have smart phones. Moreover, physical activity counseling by telephone helps sedentary people become more active. For example, a study in which health educators with bachelor's degrees counseled sedentary older adults by telephone about home-based physical activity found that telephone counseling led to better adherence to moderate- and vigorous-intensity physical activity programs than a structured exercise class did (King et al., 1988; King et al., 1991).

Another study compared the effectiveness of health educator vs. computer-automated physical activity phone counseling (King et al., 2002; King et al., 2007). In the computer-based program, participants used the touch pads on their telephones to enter their weekly minutes of activity or their intentions to become active, their activity goals for the upcoming week, and whether they wanted to hear information on relevant topics regarding physical activity. The computer system stored their data and delivered recorded voice messages that were appropriate for their stages of motivational readiness, whereas other studies have used Interactive Voice Response (IVR) systems (Brown et al., 2021) and text messaging for similar purposes (Marcus et al., 2022).

Telephone counseling programs have the advantage of providing on-the-spot support and feedback (Marcus et al., 2000; Thirumalai et al., 2022). Moreover, such systems can be programmed to proactively call people rather than waiting for people to call in, or even function bidirectionally. This allows people to call in for physical activity counseling when they feel the need, regardless of the time of day or the day of the week, while also receiving reminders and prompts (Marcus et al., 2000; Thirumalai et al., 2022). Receiving physical activity counseling any time it is needed is usually not an option when a real person delivers the counseling. Phone counseling works when delivered via a live health educator or computer-generated voice recordings, so you can select the approach that is most appropriate given the resources available in your community. Telehealth has been on the rise since the start of the COVID-19 pandemic and shows great potential in terms of addressing related physical activity declines. In fact, preliminary findings from an ongoing trial indicate that IVR-automated physical activity phone counseling at the height of the pandemic (2020-2021) improved physical activity and related psychosocial variables in underserved rural Alabama counties, which were among the hardest hit by COVID-19 (Brown et al., 2021).

Internet

According to Pew Center (Atske & Perrin, 2021) data, 93 percent of American adults now use the Internet. While Black and Hispanic adults in the United States are less likely to own a computer or have high-speed Internet at home than White adults, advances in technology have leveled the playing field. Approximately 80 percent of White, Black and Hispanic adults have internet access via a smartphone. Moreover, 70 percent of American adults are on social media, which may represent a particularly effective strategy for reaching racial and ethnic minority communities, given the slightly higher uptake in these groups. For example, 72 to 74 percent of African American and Latino adults report using Facebook, compared to 67 percent of White adults (Auxier & Anderson, 2021).

Programs such as Step Into Motion (Marcus, Lewis et al., 2007; see chapter 5 for a more detailed description), in which the participants answered stages of change questions on a website and then were given stage-relevant messages and links to other relevant stage-appropriate material, found that this delivery mode helped sedentary adults become more active at 6-month and 12-month follow-ups. Similar websites, with tailored messaging content that draws from a bank of over 300 paragraphs addressing different psychosocial and environmental factors affecting physical activity and web tools (e.g., online calendars for logging weekly physical activity and setting goals, discussion boards, information about local physical activity resources and places to be active, and tips for overcoming common barriers), have been used with great effect among underactive Latinas. Results indicated significantly greater increases in minutes per week of physical activity for the intervention group compared to the control group. Moreover, there appears to be a dose-response type relationship because website use (logins and time spent on the website) was significantly associated with intervention success (increases in min/wk of physical activity at 12 months) among Latinas (Linke et al., 2019; Marcus et al., 2015; Mendoza-Vasconez et al., 2022).

Using the web to deliver a physical activity program allows participants to get the information in which they are interested and teaches them to gather information for themselves. Email and online chat boards are avenues for providing support and encouragement from program leaders and other program participants at any time of the day or night. Whenever a person is experiencing a barrier or a lapse, help is available. Technologies such as the Internet and computerized telephone systems are not only more cost effective than face-to-face programs, but they also provide the community with better access to physical activity advice.

WORKING WITH COMMUNITY LEADERS TO REACH YOUR TARGET AUDIENCE

Another promising method for delivering community physical activity programs is through the people who have the greatest influence over the groups of people you are trying to reach (King, 1998; Odukoya et al., 2023; Pellerine et al., 2022). These influential people might include physicians, reporters, journalists, clergy, and teachers. For example, you can record a podcast or develop a credit-granting continuing education course about physical activity promotion to train physicians, nurses, psychologists, and other health professionals to deliver stage-matched physical activity counseling to their patients. Similarly, you can offer training to physical education instructors on promoting lifestyle activity by encouraging them to use relevant cognitive and behavioral strategies with their students. Politicians, members of the clergy, and other community leaders also influence public opinion and can be helpful by endorsing your program to the community (via social media and podcasts) or at least to their constituents in the community you are targeting.

> ### Stage-Specific Strategies for Community Physical Activity Programs
>
> We created the following list of intervention strategies to help you design your own community program. As we have tried to stress in this and other chapters, no one program works for everyone, so we do not provide a step-by-step program development guide. Rather, we hope you pick some of the following strategies and generate some of your own ideas so that you can create a program that addresses the needs of your target audience, your community's stage of change, any time or staffing constraints you may be working under, and your financial resources.

Stage 1: Not Thinking About Change

For this segment of the population, your goal is to help increase awareness about the

- benefits of physical activity,
- support for it in the local community, and
- acceptance of physical activity by other community members

Here are some strategies for increasing awareness and encouraging people to begin to think about the role physical activity could play in their lives.

What communication channels might you use to reach people who are not considering becoming active?

- Distribute messages (via text message, print materials, social media posts, etc.) targeted toward people who are currently not thinking about becoming more physically active.
- Work with the media to gain visibility for your messages. You might achieve this by doing the following:
  - Invite reporters, social media influencers, and bloggers to visible or newsworthy events.
  - Work with them on writing feature stories, podcasts, or sponsored posts.
  - Provide timely news releases, articles, and short videos.
  - Participate as a guest on radio or television talk shows or podcasts. Try "taking over" a popular social media account for a day.
  - Purchase radio, television, and social media advertising.
- Display key messages and your program logo on your website, social media pages, in storefront windows, on community bulletin boards, on billboard signs, and on banners strung across the main street or at major community locations.
- Design memes and bumper stickers with physical activity and health promotion messages.
- Ask utility companies, banks, physicians, and others to place promotional and educational information in their lobbies, break rooms, and other visible areas. Ask to place promotional and educational materials in the waiting rooms of hospitals and health maintenance organizations, private physicians' offices, clinics, mental health centers, and senior citizen centers.
- Ask community organizations to share this promotional information through their email lists and social media channels.

What types of information are most relevant to people in this earliest stage?

- Host health fairs that include exercise testing, blood pressure screenings, or body fat composition assessments. Relate how these are affected by physical activity.
- Emphasize the short-term benefits of being active (e.g., feeling invigorated, sleeping better, reducing stress, feeling better about oneself) rather than the long-term benefits that these people might believe are unattainable.
- Dispel misconceptions about physical activity (e.g., "no pain, no gain," overestimated risk of injuries such as a heart attack).
- Increase awareness of what they might miss by choosing not to be active (e.g., enjoyment from being active, better self-esteem).

What are some other strategies that might move these people closer to considering change?

- Help people to visualize success—to visualize a happy, healthy, and active lifestyle.
- Encourage these people to read or think about how physical activity might benefit them. For this group, it is better to focus on the benefits of physical activity and not dwell on the risks of a sedentary lifestyle.
- Link the benefits of a physically active lifestyle to people's highest priorities and values in life (e.g., relationships with family, personal faith, health, or happiness).
- Encourage these people to see how their sedentary behavior affects them and others in their lives (e.g., sedentary parents model an unhealthy lifestyle for their children).

How might you show community support for physical activity?

- Encourage health care providers to advise their patients on how they might benefit from physical activity.
- Choose a spokesperson that the target audience trusts, respects, believes, or can identify with to help increase awareness. Identify role models within the community. Recruit local people to endorse your program.
- Conduct targeted informational campaigns and sessions, such as the following:
  - Lunch-'n'-learn or community lectures
  - Workshops, seminars, or adult education classes
  - Youth group programs
  - One-on-one counseling or instruction
  - Guest talk-show appearances on television, radio, and podcasts
  - Featured articles in newspapers and websites
- Provide informative webinars for worksites, schools, and community organizations.

Stage 2: Thinking About Change

For this segment of the community, one of your goals is to increase awareness of the benefits of physical activity, community support, and the social norms for this behavior. Another goal is to move these people closer to actually trying the behavior. Here are some ideas for achieving these goals.

What communication channels might you use?

- Distribute information targeted toward people who are thinking about becoming more physically active or include health and physical activity tips in general publications.

- Increase awareness by working with the media to gain visibility for your messages:
    - Invite bloggers and reporters to visible or newsworthy events.
    - Work with reporters on writing feature stories and social media content.
    - Provide timely news releases or newspaper articles.
    - Participate as a guest on radio or television talk shows or podcasts.
    - Purchase radio, television, social media advertisements.
- Display key messages and your program logo online, in storefront windows, on community bulletin boards, on billboard signs, and on banners strung across the main street or at major community locations.
- Design bumper stickers with physical activity and health promotion messages.
- Ask utility companies, banks, physicians, and others to place promotional and educational information in their monthly billings and "share" related social media posts.
- Ask to place promotional and educational materials in the waiting rooms of hospitals and health maintenance organizations, private physicians' offices, clinics, mental health centers, and senior citizen centers.
- Make health videos available online.
- Create a website with links to relevant, stage-appropriate physical activity and health sites.

What types of information are most relevant to people who are considering becoming more active?

- Provide basic information about what is needed to achieve a physically active lifestyle, such as selecting the appropriate shoes or clothing.
- Describe a variety of activities available to most people that can be done alone or with family and friends.
- Suggest ways to build some activity into one's daily routine (e.g., taking the stairs at work).
- Dispel misconceptions about physical activity (e.g., "no pain, no gain," overestimated risk of injury such as a heart attack).

What are some other strategies that might move these people closer to trying some physical activity?

- Provide messages that link physical activity to values or issues relevant to your target audience.
- Help them weigh the pros and cons of a physically active lifestyle. Focus on the costs of changing (effort, energy, and the things they must give up to overcome a sedentary lifestyle) and how they might manage them.
- Encourage them to start off slowly (e.g., a 5- or 10-minute walk) and build gradually (add 5 min/day/wk) and explain how to reward themselves when they achieve their goals.

- Distribute self-assessment questionnaires such as the Physical Activity Readiness Questionnaire (found in chapter 7) and the decisional balance questionnaire (questionnaire 4.4 in appendix A).
- Help people to visualize success—to visualize a happy, healthy, and active lifestyle.

How might you show community support for trying some physical activity?

- Host health fairs that include exercise testing, blood pressure screenings, or body fat composition assessments. Relate how these are affected by physical activity.
- Choose a spokesperson that the target audience trusts, respects, believes, or can identify with. Identify role models within the community. Recruit local people to endorse your program.
- Encourage health care providers to advise these patients on how they might benefit from physical activity and some steps they could take to begin a physically active lifestyle.
- Conduct targeted informational campaigns and sessions (USDHHS et al., 1999), such as the following:
  - Lunch-'n'-learn or community lectures
  - Workshops, webinars, or adult education classes
  - Youth group programs
  - One-on-one counseling or instruction
  - Guest talk-show appearances on television, radio, and podcasts
  - Featured articles in newspapers and websites
- Give informative presentations at worksites, in schools, and to community organizations such as Rotary Clubs.
- Create automated physical activity hotlines and websites that people can contact for information about physical activity.

Stage 3: Doing Some Physical Activity

People in this stage are likely to be receptive to physical activity messages because they are doing some activity but not enough to meet national guidelines. Therefore, your goal for this group is to encourage them to increase the amount of physical activity they do each week. To accomplish this goal, you might choose to do some of the following.

What communication channels might you use to reach these people?

- Distribute materials targeted toward people who want to become more physically active.
- Develop or make available self-instructional materials, such as video tutorials, how-to guides, manuals, and kits.
- Provide formal and informal activity-oriented instructional programs, such as workshops, classes, webinars, demonstrations, lessons, and lectures.

- Sponsor "meet the expert" events (both online and face to face) so community members can learn directly from those who have mastered various skills.
- Create hotlines and websites that people can contact with questions about physical activity.
- Make a website and social media account with links to relevant physical activity and health sites.

What types of information are most relevant to people who need to increase their level of physical activity?

- Discuss how to develop a plan for regular activity.
- Provide ideas for making activity more fun.
- Teach methods of self-monitoring to keep track of progress.
- Discuss barriers to physical activity and ways to overcome them.
- Suggest ways people might restructure their environments to increase the possibility that they will be active (e.g., keep walking shoes at work or by the door at home).
- Discuss ways to use exercise or sports equipment properly and safely.
- Describe stretching, warm-up, and cool-down techniques.

What are some other strategies that might move these people closer to meeting national guidelines for regular activity?

- Host health and fitness fairs and online events that include exercise testing to demonstrate that each person needs more physical activity.
- Emphasize small, specific, and realistic goals.
- Encourage the use of self-rewards for meeting goals.
- Encourage people to make use of social support networks such as walking clubs or friends or coworkers who exercise during lunch breaks.
- Suggest exercising while sitting in a chair, standing, or watching television.
- Start a walking or jogging program.

How might you show community support for increasing physical activity?

- Develop a community resource list so that people will know where to find courses or opportunities to develop skills.
- Appeal to the community's competitive spirit with step contests, prizes, incentives, publicity, recognition, rewards, and fun promotional items.
- Establish competitive programs among individuals, neighborhoods, churches, organizations, or businesses.
- Incentives might include discounts at recreational facilities, fitness club memberships, sports or exercise equipment or apparel, a free lunch, a book, a T-shirt, a pair of walking shoes, public recognition, and community awards.

- Encourage health care providers to advise their patients to increase their levels of physical activity and to take advantage of the many community resources you can identify.
- Provide opportunities to try various types of physical activity for just one day or one event.
  - Community walking events
  - Using the stairs instead of elevators for one day or one week
  - Bicycle-to-work day or other bicycling events
  - Periodic fun runs
  - Lunchtime walking groups at local businesses, schools, or shopping malls
  - Trial memberships and guest passes to use recreational facilities
- For groups of various ages or levels of experience, work with physical education instructors, physical therapists, or exercise physiologists to design appropriate and quality instructional programs.

Stage 4: Doing Enough Physical Activity

These people have recently become active at the level recommended by national guidelines. Your goal is to foster continued participation in physical activity and to bolster continued community support for activity. To accomplish this, you can do some of the following.

What communication channels might you use to reach regularly active people?

- Distribute information targeted toward people who are physically active at the level recommended by national guidelines but at risk for relapse.
- Establish telephone hotlines that people can call or text with questions about physical activity.
- Develop a community resource list or website so that people will know where to find courses or opportunities to develop new skills.
- Sponsor "meet the expert" events so that community members can learn directly from those who have mastered various skills.
- Create a website and social media accounts with links to relevant physical activity and health sites.

What types of information are most relevant to people who are regularly active?

- Provide a list of activities that will reduce the risk of injury and boredom and encourage people to try different activities.
- Describe stretching, warm-up, and cool-down techniques.

- Suggest ways to restructure their environment (e.g., keep walking shoes at work or by the door at home) to increase the possibility that they will choose an active pursuit rather than a sedentary one.
- Instruct on how to avoid the risk of injury from exercise.
- Teach self-monitoring methods for keeping track of progress.

What are some other strategies to help these people stay active?

- Encourage the use of social support networks such as walking clubs or friends or coworkers who exercise during lunch breaks.
- Instruct on how to anticipate lapses and accept them as a normal part of the change process so that the occasional lapse is not viewed as a failure.
- Help identify situations that are more likely to lead to a lapse and develop a plan for staying active in these situations.
- Encourage these people to build in rewards to maintain motivation. These can be tangible, such as a new pair of walking shoes, or intangible, such as making a mental note of achieving a goal.
- Help these people develop long-term goals (e.g., participating in a 5k fun walk in a few months) and short-term goals to help reach their long-term goals (e.g., increasing the distance walked by half a mile [0.8 km] per week).

How might you show community support for staying physically active at nationally recommended levels?

- Appeal to the community's competitive spirit with step contests, prizes, incentives, publicity, recognition, rewards, and fun promotional items. Establish competitive programs among individuals, neighborhoods, churches, organizations, or businesses. Incentives might include discounts at recreational facilities, fitness club memberships, sports or exercise equipment or apparel, a free lunch, a book, a T-shirt, a pair of walking shoes, public recognition, and community awards.
- Encourage health care providers to ask their patients about physical activity and tell their patients about community resources for physical activity.
- Provide opportunities to try different types of physical activity for just one day or one event:
  - Community walking events
  - Using stairs instead of elevators for one day or one week
  - Bicycle-to-work day or other bicycling events
  - Periodic fun walks or runs
  - Lunchtime walking groups at local businesses, schools, or shopping malls
  - Trial memberships and guest passes to use recreational facilities

Stage 5: Making Physical Activity a Habit

People in this group are familiar with physical activity because they have been regularly active for at least six months. Your goal is to help them stay active by anticipating lapses, planning for situations that jeopardize their activity, and keeping them motivated over the long term. Here are some suggestions for achieving these goals.

What communication channels might you use to reach regularly active people?

- Distribute information targeted toward people who are active and have been for at least six months.
- Create telephone hotlines that people can call or text with questions about physical activity or activity-related injuries.
- Develop a community resource list so that people will know where to find courses or opportunities to develop new activity skills.
- Sponsor "meet the expert" events so community members can learn directly from those who have mastered various skills that may be new to these people.

What types of information are most relevant to people in this stage?

- Teach how to anticipate lapses and accept them as a normal part of the change process so that the occasional lapse is not viewed as a failure.
- Help people identify situations likely to lead to lapses and encourage them to develop plans for staying active in these situations.
- Remind regularly active people to build in rewards to maintain motivation. These can be tangible, such as a new pair of walking shoes, or intangible, such as making a mental note of achieving a goal.
- Provide a list of activities that will reduce the risk of injury and boredom, and encourage them to try different activities.

What are some other strategies to help these people stay active?

- Encourage the use of social support networks such as walking clubs or friends or coworkers who exercise during lunch breaks.
- Help people recognize and appreciate their personal responsibility for maintaining change.
- Suggest how these people might serve as role models for others.

How might you show community support for the maintenance of regular physical activity?

- Appeal to the community's competitive spirit with step contests, prizes, incentives, publicity, recognition, rewards, and fun promotional items.

- Establish competitive programs among individuals, neighborhoods, churches, organizations, or businesses.
- Incentives might include discounts at recreational facilities, fitness club memberships, sports or exercise equipment or apparel, a free lunch, a book, a T-shirt, a pair of walking shoes, public recognition, and community awards.
- Encourage health care providers to ask their patients about physical activity and counsel them on relapse prevention.
- Provide opportunities to try different types of physical activity for just one day or one event:
  - Community walking events
  - Using stairs instead of elevators for one day or one week
  - Bicycle-to-work day or other bicycling events
  - Periodic fun walks or runs
  - Lunchtime walking groups at local businesses, schools, or shopping malls
  - Trial memberships and guest passes to use recreational facilities

CONCLUSION

When addressing physical activity at a community level, "one size fits all" may fit none. For best results, you will likely need to spend some time getting to know the community, determining your target audience, assessing their physical activity needs and perceptions, and their resources and barriers. There may be factors influencing physical activity at many levels (neighborhood walkability, access to safe local parks, etc.). We describe methods for ascertaining how the built environment supports or inhibits physical activity in the community and using these insights to guide your approach. Examples from social marketing are provided as a useful framework for considering what types of messages to deliver and how you will deliver your program. Once it is time to put your program together, the strategies you select should be based on the scale of your project and the funds available. We provide tips on tailoring and targeting your physical activity messages for enhanced relevance and appeal to the community. The Stage-Specific Strategies section offers some suggestions for print and online materials, media coverage, and community events based on your target audience's motivational readiness for changing their physical activity behavior. You can use these and your own ideas to improve physical activity participation in your community.

APPENDIX A

QUESTIONNAIRES

This book's focus was to translate theories and concepts from behavioral science research into a handbook useful for health professionals who are involved in planning, developing, implementing, or evaluating physical activity programs. Questionnaires can be a valuable tool for those health professionals who are undertaking such roles. In the following pages, please find the questionnaires referenced throughout the book. Copy them and use them to help you develop effective physical activity interventions. (For more detailed information about scoring these questionnaires, please see chapter 4.)

Questionnaire 2.1:	Physical Activity Stages of Change	176
Questionnaire 2.2:	Actividad Física – Etapas de Cambio	177
Questionnaire 4.1:	Processes of Change	178
Questionnaire 4.2:	Confidence (Self-Efficacy)	181
Questionnaire 4.3:	Social Support for Physical Activity Scale	182
Questionnaire 4.4:	Decisional Balance	183
Questionnaire 4.5:	Outcome Expectations for Exercise	185
Questionnaire 4.6:	Physical Activity Enjoyment Scale	186
Questionnaire 7.1:	Physical Activity History	187

QUESTIONNAIRE 2.1
PHYSICAL ACTIVITY STAGES OF CHANGE

For each of the following questions, please circle Yes or No. Please be sure to read the questions carefully.

Physical activity or exercise includes activities such as walking briskly, jogging, bicycling, swimming, or any other activity in which the exertion is at least as intense as these activities.

	No	Yes
1. I am currently physically active.	0	1
2. I intend to become more physically active in the next 6 months.	0	1

For activity to be *regular*, it must add up to a *total* of 30 minutes or more per day and be done at least five days per week. For example, you could take one 30-minute walk or take three 10-minute walks for a daily total of 30 minutes.

	No	Yes
3. I currently engage in *regular* physical activity.	0	1
4. I have been *regularly* physically active for the past 6 months.	0	1

Note: You may want to cover the following scoring algorithm before reproducing this questionnaire for a client.

Scoring Algorithm

If (question 1 = 0 and question 2 = 0), then you are at stage 1.

If (question 1 = 0 and question 2 = 1), then you are at stage 2.

If (question 1 = 1 and question 3 = 0), then you are at stage 3.

If (question 1 = 1, question 3 = 1, and question 4 = 0), then you are at stage 4.

If (question 1 = 1, question 3 = 1, and question 4 = 1), then you are at stage 5.

From B. Marcus and D. Pekmezi, *Motivating People to Be Physically Active,* 3rd ed. (Champaign, IL: Human Kinetics, 2025). Reprinted by permission, from B.H. Marcus et al., "The Stages and Processes of Exercise Adoption and Maintenance in a Worksite Sample," *Health Psychology* 11 (1992): 386-395.

QUESTIONNAIRE 2.2
ACTIVIDAD FÍSICA – ETAPAS DE CAMBIO

INSTRUCCIONES: Por favor conteste las siguientes preguntas acerca de usted misma.

	No	Si
1. Actualmente yo hago ejercicios	N	S
2. Tengo la intención de hacer más ejercicios en los próximos 6 meses.	N	S

Para que la actividad física sea regular, tiene que acumular un total de 150 minutos a la semana. Por ejemplo, podría tomar una caminata de 30 minutos, 5 días de la semana. Durante esta actividad su corazón se agita y su respiración se acelera.

	No	Si
1. Actualmente yo hago actividad física regularmente de por lo menos 30 minutos por día y por lo menos 5 días de la semana.	N	S
2. Yo he hecho actividad física regularmente (en forma continua) durante los últimos 6 meses.	N	S

Date: _____ ID: _____ Session: _____

From B. Marcus and D. Pekmezi, *Motivating People to Be Physically Active*, 3rd ed. (Champaign, IL: Human Kinetics, 2025).

QUESTIONNAIRE 4.1
PROCESSES OF CHANGE

Physical activity or exercise includes activities such as walking briskly, jogging, bicycling, swimming, and any other activity in which the exertion is at least as intense as these activities.

The following experiences can affect the exercise habits of some people. Think of any similar behaviors you may currently have or have had during the past month. Then rate how frequently the behavior occurs. Please circle the number that best describes your answer for each experience.

How frequently does this occur?

1 = never

2 = seldom

3 = occasionally

4 = often

5 = repeatedly

1. Instead of remaining inactive, I engage in some physical activity.
   1 2 3 4 5
2. I tell myself I am able to be physically active if I want to.
   1 2 3 4 5
3. I put things around my home to remind me to be physically active.
   1 2 3 4 5
4. I tell myself that if I try hard enough, I can be physically active.
   1 2 3 4 5
5. I recall information people have personally given me on the benefits of physical activity.
   1 2 3 4 5
6. I make commitments to be physically active.
   1 2 3 4 5
7. I reward myself when I am physically active.
   1 2 3 4 5
8. I think about information from articles and advertisements on how to make physical activity a regular part of my life.
   1 2 3 4 5
9. I keep things around my place of work that remind me to be physically active.
   1 2 3 4 5
10. I find society changing in ways that make it easier to be physically active.
    1 2 3 4 5

11. Warnings about the health hazards of inactivity affect me emotionally.
    1 2 3 4 5
12. Dramatic portrayals of the evils of inactivity affect me emotionally.
    1 2 3 4 5
13. I react emotionally to warnings about an inactive lifestyle.
    1 2 3 4 5
14. I worry that inactivity can be harmful to my body.
    1 2 3 4 5
15. I am considering the idea that regular physical activity would make me a healthier, happier person to be around.
    1 2 3 4 5
16. I have someone I can depend on when I am having problems with physical activity.
    1 2 3 4 5
17. I read articles about physical activity in an attempt to learn more about it.
    1 2 3 4 5
18. I try to set realistic physical activity goals for myself rather than set myself up for failure by expecting too much.
    1 2 3 4 5
19. I have a healthy friend who encourages me to be physically active when I don't feel up to it.
    1 2 3 4 5
20. When I am physically active, I tell myself that I am being good to myself by taking care of my body.
    1 2 3 4 5
21. The time I spend being physically active is my special time to relax and recover from the day's worries, not a task to get out of the way.
    1 2 3 4 5
22. I am aware of more and more people encouraging me to be physically active these days.
    1 2 3 4 5
23. I do something nice for myself for making efforts to be more physically active.
    1 2 3 4 5
24. I have someone who points out my rationalizations for not being physically active.
    1 2 3 4 5
25. I have someone who provides feedback about my physical activity.
    1 2 3 4 5

(continued)

Questionnaire 4.1 Processes of Change *(continued)*

26. I remove things that contribute to my inactivity.
    1 2 3 4 5
27. I am the only one responsible for my health, and only I can decide whether or not I will be physically active.
    1 2 3 4 5
28. I look for information related to physical activity.
    1 2 3 4 5
29. I avoid spending long periods of time in environments that promote inactivity.
    1 2 3 4 5
30. I feel that I would be a better role model for others if I were regularly physically active.
    1 2 3 4 5
31. I think about the type of person I would be if I were physically active.
    1 2 3 4 5
32. I notice that more businesses are encouraging their employees to be physically active by offering fitness courses and time off to work out.
    1 2 3 4 5
33. I wonder how my inactivity affects those people who are close to me.
    1 2 3 4 5
34. I realize that I might be able to influence others to be healthier if I would be more physically active.
    1 2 3 4 5
35. I get frustrated with myself when I am not physically active.
    1 2 3 4 5
36. I am aware that many health clubs now provide babysitting services to their members.
    1 2 3 4 5
37. Some of my close friends might be more physically active if I were.
    1 2 3 4 5
38. I consider the fact that I would feel more confident in myself if I were regularly physically active.
    1 2 3 4 5
39. When I feel tired, I make myself be physically active anyway because I know I will feel better afterward.
    1 2 3 4 5
40. When I'm feeling tense, I find physical activity a great way to relieve my worries.
    1 2 3 4 5

From B. Marcus and D. Pekmezi, *Motivating People to Be Physically Active*, 3rd ed. (Champaign, IL: Human Kinetics, 2025). Reprinted by permission from B.H. Marcus et al., "The Stages and Processes of Exercise Adoption and Maintenance in a Worksite Sample," *Health Psychology* 11 (1992): 386-395.

QUESTIONNAIRE 4.2
CONFIDENCE (SELF-EFFICACY)

Physical activity or exercise includes activities such as walking briskly, jogging, bicycling, swimming, and any other activity in which the exertion is at least as intense as these activities.

Circle the number that indicates how confident you are that you could be physically active in each of the following situations:

Scale

1 = not at all confident
2 = slightly confident
3 = moderately confident
4 = very confident
5 = extremely confident

1. When I am tired	1	2	3	4	5
2. When I am in a bad mood	1	2	3	4	5
3. When I feel I don't have time	1	2	3	4	5
4. When I am on vacation	1	2	3	4	5
5. When it is raining or snowing	1	2	3	4	5

From B. Marcus and D. Pekmezi, *Motivating People to Be Physically Active,* 3rd ed. (Champaign, IL: Human Kinetics, 2025). Reprinted with permission from B.H. Marcus, V.C. Selby, R.S. Niaura, and J.S. Rossi, "Self-Efficacy and the Stages of Exercise Behavior Change," *Research Quarterly for Exercise and Sport,* 63, no. 1 (1992): 60-66. Copyright 1992 by the American Alliance for Health, Physical Education, Recreation and Dance, 1900 Association Drive, Reston, VA 20191, reprinted by permission of the publisher (Taylor & Francis Ltd, http://www.tandfonline.com).

QUESTIONNAIRE 4.3
SOCIAL SUPPORT FOR PHYSICAL ACTIVITY SCALE

The following questions refer to social support for your physical activity.

The following is a list of things people might do or say to someone who is trying to do physical activity regularly. Please read and answer every question. If you are not physically active, then some of the questions may not apply to you.

Please rate each question *twice*. Under "Family," rate how often anyone living in your household has said or done what is described during the past 3 months. Under "Friends," rate how often your friends, acquaintances, or coworkers have said or done what is described during the past 3 months.

Please write *one* number from the following rating scale in each space:

1 = none
2 = rarely
3 = a few times
4 = often
5 = very often
0 = does not apply

	Family	Friends
1. Did physical activities with me		
2. Offered to do physical activities with me		
3. Gave me helpful reminders to be physically active (e.g., "Are you going to do your activity tonight?")		
4. Gave me encouragement to stick with my activity program		
5. Changed their schedule so we could do physical activities together		
6. Discussed physical activity with me		
7. Complained about the time I spend doing physical activity		
8. Criticized me or made fun of me for doing physical activities		
9. Gave me rewards for being physically active (e.g., gave me something I liked)		
10. Planned for physical activities on recreational outings		
11. Helped plan events around my physical activities		
12. Asked me for ideas on how they can be more physically active		
13. Talked about how much they like to do physical activity		

From B. Marcus and D. Pekmezi, *Motivating People to Be Physically Active,* 3rd ed. (Champaign, IL: Human Kinetics, 2025). Reprinted by permission from J.F. Sallis et al., "The Development of Scales to Measure Social Support for Diet and Exercise Behaviors," *Preventive Medicine* 16 (1987): 825-836, copyright 1987, with permission from Elsevier.

QUESTIONNAIRE 4.4
DECISIONAL BALANCE

Physical activity or exercise includes activities such as walking briskly, jogging, bicycling, swimming, and any other activity in which the exertion is at least as intense as these activities.

Please rate how important each of these statements is in your decision of whether to be physically active. In each case, think about how you feel right now, not how you have felt in the past or would like to feel.

Scale

1 = not at all important
2 = slightly important
3 = moderately important
4 = very important
5 = extremely important

1. I would have more energy for my family and friends if I were regularly physically active.
   1 2 3 4 5

2. Regular physical activity would help me relieve tension.
   1 2 3 4 5

3. I think I would be too tired to do my daily work after being physically active.
   1 2 3 4 5

4. I would feel more confident if I were regularly physically active.
   1 2 3 4 5

5. I would sleep more soundly if I were regularly physically active.
   1 2 3 4 5

6. I would feel good about myself if I kept my commitment to be regularly physically active.
   1 2 3 4 5

7. I would find it difficult to find a physical activity that I enjoy and that is not affected by bad weather.
   1 2 3 4 5

8. I would like my body better if I were regularly physically active.
   1 2 3 4 5

9. It would be easier for me to perform routine physical tasks if I were regularly physically active.
   1 2 3 4 5

10. I would feel less stressed if I were regularly physically active.
    1 2 3 4 5

(continued)

Questionnaire 4.4 Decisional Balance *(continued)*

11. I feel uncomfortable when I am physically active because I get out of breath and my heart beats very fast.
    1 2 3 4 5

12. I would feel more comfortable with my body if I were regularly physically active.
    1 2 3 4 5

13. Regular physical activity would take too much of my time.
    1 2 3 4 5

14. Regular physical activity would help me have a more positive outlook on life.
    1 2 3 4 5

15. I would have less time for my family and friends if I were regularly physically active.
    1 2 3 4 5

16. At the end of the day, I am too exhausted to be physically active.
    1 2 3 4 5

From B. Marcus and D. Pekmezi, *Motivating People to Be Physically Active,* 3rd ed. (Champaign, IL: Human Kinetics, 2025). Reprinted by permission from B.H. Marcus, W. Rakowski, and J.S. Rossi, "Assessing Motivational Readiness and Decision-Making for Exercise," *Health Psychology* 11(1992): 257-261.

QUESTIONNAIRE 4.5
OUTCOME EXPECTATIONS FOR EXERCISE

The following are statements about the benefits of exercise (walking, jogging, swimming, biking, stretching, or lifting weights). Circle the number representing the degree to which you agree or disagree with these statements.

1. Makes me feel better physically
   1   2   3   4   5

2. Makes my mood better in general
   1   2   3   4   5

3. Helps me feel less tired
   1   2   3   4   5

4. Makes my muscles stronger
   1   2   3   4   5

5. Is an activity I enjoy doing
   1   2   3   4   5

6. Gives me a sense of personal accomplishment
   1   2   3   4   5

7. Makes me more alert mentally
   1   2   3   4   5

8. Improves my endurance in performing my daily activities (such as personal care, cooking, shopping, light cleaning, taking out garbage)
   1   2   3   4   5

9. Helps to strengthen my bones
   1   2   3   4   5

From B. Marcus and D. Pekmezi, *Motivating People to Be Physically Active,* 3rd ed. (Champaign, IL: Human Kinetics, 2025). Reprinted by permission from B. Resnick et al., "Outcome Expectations for Exercise Scale: Utility and Psychometrics," *Journal of Gerontology: Social Sciences* 55B (2000): S352-S356.

QUESTIONNAIRE 4.6
PHYSICAL ACTIVITY ENJOYMENT SCALE

Please rate how you feel at the moment about physical activity. Below is a list of feelings with respect to physical activity. For each feeling, please mark the number that best describes you.

	1	2	3	4	5	6	7	
1. I enjoy it.								I hate it.
2. I feel bored.								I feel interested.
3. I dislike it.								I like it.
4. I find it pleasurable.								I find it unpleasurable.
5. I am very absorbed in physical activity.								I am not at all absorbed in physical activity.
6. It's no fun at all.								It's a lot of fun.
7. I find it energizing.								I find it tiring.
8. It makes me depressed.								It makes me happy.
9. It's very pleasant.								It's very unpleasant.
10. I feel good physically while doing it.								I feel bad physically while doing it.
11. It's very invigorating.								It's not at all invigorating.
12. I am very frustrated by it.								I am not at all frustrated by it.
13. It's very gratifying.								It's not at all gratifying.
14. It's very exhilarating.								It's not at all exhilarating.
15. It's not at all stimulating.								It's very stimulating.
16. It gives me a strong sense of accomplishment.								It does not give me any sense of accomplishment.
17. It's very refreshing.								It's not at all refreshing.
18. I would rather be doing something else.								There is nothing else I would rather be doing.

From B. Marcus and D. Pekmezi, *Motivating People to Be Physically Active*, 3rd ed. (Champaign, IL: Human Kinetics, 2025). Adapted by permission from D. Kendzierski and K.J. DeCarlo, "Physical Activity Enjoyment Scale: Two Validation Studies," *Journal of Sport & Exercise Psychology* 13, no. 1 (1991): 62-63.

QUESTIONNAIRE 7.1
PHYSICAL ACTIVITY HISTORY

If you do *not* currently participate in physical activity, answer these questions:

1. How long has it been since you did *regular* physical activity or exercise?
    a. Less than 6 months
    b. More than 6 months but less than 1 year
    c. More than 1 year but less than 2 years
    d. More than 2 years but less than 5 years
    e. More than 5 years but less than 10 years
    f. More than 10 years
    g. I have never been regularly physically active.

If you are *currently* physically active, answer the following questions:

1. How many days per week are you physically active? _____.
2. Approximately how many minutes are you physically active each time? _____.
3. How long have you been physically active at this level? _____.
4. What activities do you do? _____.

Answer the following questions whether or not you are currently physically active.

1. As an adult, were there ever times when you were physically active regularly for at least 3 months and then stopped being physically active for at least 3 months?
    a. Yes
    b. No
2. If yes, how many times? _____.
3. Regarding the most recent time, why did you stop your activity? (Please check as many as apply.)

Lack of time because of

_____ Work or school	_____ Lack of physical activity partner
_____ Household duties	_____ Lack of interest in physical activity
_____ Children	_____ Health problems
_____ Social activities	_____ Injury
_____ Spouse	_____ Season or weather change
_____ Lack of money	_____ Personal stress
_____ Lack of facilities	_____ Other: _____

From B. Marcus and D. Pekmezi, *Motivating People to Be Physically Active*, 3rd ed. (Champaign, IL: Human Kinetics, 2025).

APPENDIX B

RESOURCES

The following is a list of organizations, suggested readings, and helpful websites you can use to enhance your programs.

ORGANIZATIONS

American College of Sports Medicine (ACSM)
www.acsm.org

American Heart Association National Center
www.heart.org

Center for Behavioral and Preventive Medicine
www.lifespan.org/centers-services/center-behavioral-and-preventive-medicine

Centers for Disease Control and Prevention (CDC)
www.cdc.gov/nccdphp/dnpa

The Cooper Institute
www.cooperinstitute.org

Stanford Prevention Research Center (SPRC)
https://prevention.stanford.edu

Human Kinetics
www.HumanKinetics.com

National Heart, Lung, and Blood Institute (NHLBI)
www.nhlbi.nih.gov

President's Council on Sports, Fitness, and Nutrition (PCSFN)
https://health.gov/pcsfn

International Society of Physical Activity and Health
https://ispah.org/

World Health Organization
https://www.who.int/health-topics/physical-activity#tab=tab_1

Canadian Society for Exercise Physiology
https://csepguidelines.ca/

SUGGESTED READING

Sylvia LG, Bernstein EE, Hubbard JL, Keating L, Anderson EJ. Practical guide to measuring physical activity. J Acad Nutr Diet. 2014 Feb;114(2):199-208. doi: 10.1016/j.jand.2013.09.018. Epub 2013 Nov 28. PMID: 24290836; PMCID: PMC3915355.

A collection of physical activity questionnaires for health-related research. (1997). *Medicine and Science in Sports and Exercise, 29*(Suppl. 6).

American College of Sports Medicine. (1995). *Guidelines for exercise testing and prescription* (5th ed.). Williams & Wilkins.

Blair, S.N., Dunn, A.L., Marcus, B.H., Carpenter, R.A., & Jaret, P. (2001). *Active Living Every Day: 20 Weeks to Lifelong Vitality.* Human Kinetics.

Bouchard, C., Shephard, R., & Stephens, T. (1993). *Physical activity, fitness, and health: International proceedings and consensus statement.* Human Kinetics.

Centers for Disease Control. (1999). *Promoting physical activity: A guide for community action.* Human Kinetics.

Measurement of physical activity [Special issue]. (2000). *Research Quarterly for Exercise and Sport, 71.*

WEB SITES

Move More Together, American Heart Association: www.heart.org/en/healthy-living/fitness/fitness-basics/move-more-together

- *Information:* How to find target heart rate, how to exercise safely
- *Assessment:* Fitness level, BMI, target heart rate
- *Strategies for change:* Self-monitoring, goal setting

SHAPE America: www.shapeamerica.org

- *Information:* Fitness glossary, physical activity IQ test
- *Assessment:* Fitness, strength, aerobic fitness
- *Strategies for change:* Benefits of physical activity, overcoming barriers

Mayo Clinic Fitness and Sports Medicine Center: www.mayoclinic.com/health/fitness/SM99999

- *Information:* How to plan and start an exercise program, budgeting costs, strength training and stretching tips, injury prevention, sample walking programs
- *Assessment:* Fitness level, fitness awareness, BMI
- *Strategies for change:* Benefits of physical activity, overcoming barriers

American Academy of Family Physicians: http://familydoctor.org

- *Information:* How to plan and start an exercise program, injury prevention, aerobic exercise, weight training
- *Assessment:* Target heart rate
- *Strategies for change:* Self-monitoring, social support, relapse prevention

American Council on Exercise: www.acefitness.org/aboutace

- *Information:* Safe and effective ways to exercise
- *Strategies for change:* Benefits of physical activity < sb3list > ACSM Health and Fitness Information: www.acsm.org/health%2Bfitness/index.htm
- *Information:* Active aging tips, guidelines for aerobic activity and getting started with exercise
- *Assessment:* Target heart rate
- *Strategies for change:* Social support

Chapter 1
https://health.gov/our-work/nutrition-physical-activity/physical-activity-guidelines/current-guidelines

Chapter 2
The Transtheoretical Model: https://web.uri.edu/cprc/transtheoretical-model

Chapter 3
Theory at a glance: A guide for health promotion practice
https://cancercontrol.cancer.gov/sites/default/files/2020-06/theory.pdf

Chapter 4
Rhodes, Ryan E., Boudreau, Patrick, Joselsson, Karin, & Iversson, Andreas (2019). Mediators of physical activity behavior change interventions among adults: A systematic review and meta-analysis. *Health Psychology Review*, https://pubmed.ncbi.nlm.nih.gov/31875768/

Chapter 5
Johnson, S. S. (2013). Building motivation: How ready are you? In Nigg, C. (Ed.), *ACSM's Behavioral Aspects of Physical Activity and Exercise*. (Point (Lippincott Williams & Wilkins)), 103-128 , https://cme.lww.com/files/BuildingMotivationHowReadyAreYou-1550445822749.pdf

Ma, J. K., Floegel, T.A., Li, L. C., Leese, J., De Vera, M. A., Beauchamp, M. R., Taunton, J., Liu-Ambrose, T., Allen, K. D. (2021). Tailored physical activity behavior change interventions: Challenges and opportunities. *Transl Behav Med.* 11(12), 2174-2181. https://www.ncbi.nlm.nih.gov/pmc/articles/PMC8672936/

Joseph, R., Keller, C., Affuso, O., & Ainsworth, B. (2017). Designing culturally relevant physical activity programs for African-American women: A framework for intervention development. *Journal of Racial and Ethnic Health Disparities*, 4(3), 397-409. https://link.springer.com/article/10.1007/s40615-016-0240-1

Chapter 6

Rikli, R. E., & Jones, C. J. (1999). Functional fitness normative scores for community residing older adults ages 60-94. *Journal of Aging and Physical Activity*, 7, 160-179.

Ferguson, Ty, et al. (2022). Effectiveness of wearable activity trackers to increase physical activity and improve health: A systematic review of systematic reviews and meta-analyses. *The Lancet Digital Health*, 4(8), 615-626. https://doi.org/10.1016/S2589-7500(22)00111-X.

Chapter 7

Swann, Christiaan, Jackman, P. C., et al. (2023). The (over)use of SMART goals for physical activity promotion: A narrative review and critique, *Health Psychology Review*, 17:2, 211-226. https://www.tandfonline.com/doi/full/10.1080/17437199.2021.2023608

Chapter 8

Wittingham, Martyn, & Martin, Jennifer. (2020). How to do group therapy using telehealth. https://www.apaservices.org/practice/legal/technology/group-therapy-telehealth-covid-19

Health and Human Services. (n.d.). *Telehealth for behavioral health care.* https://telehealth.hhs.gov/providers/best-practice-guides/telehealth-for-behavioral-health/group-teletherapy

Chapter 9

The role of employers in improving the health of their employees. https://www.cdc.gov/physicalactivity/activepeoplehealthynation/everyone-can-be-involved/employers.html

Merom, D., Stanaway, F., Gebel, K., Sweeting, J., Tiedemann, A., Mumu, S., Ding, D. (2021). Supporting active ageing before retirement: a systematic review and meta-analysis of workplace physical activity interventions targeting older employees. *BMJ Open*. Jun 30;11(6): https://bmjopen.bmj.com/content/11/6/e045818

Chapter 10

Xia, Y., Deshpande, S., Bonates, T. (2016). Effectiveness of social marketing interventions to promote physical activity among adults: A systematic review. *J Phys Act Health*. 13(11), 1263-1274. https://pubmed.ncbi.nlm.nih.gov/27633626

Ma, J. K., Floegel, T. A., Li, L. C., Leese, J., De Vera, M. A., Beauchamp, M. R., Taunton, J., Liu-Ambrose, T., Allen. K. D. (2021). Tailored physical activity behavior change interventions: challenges and opportunities. *Transl Behav Med*. 11(12), 2174-2181. https://www.ncbi.nlm.nih.gov/pmc/articles/PMC8672936/

REFERENCES

Chapter 1

Caspersen, C.J. (1989). Physical activity epidemiology: Concepts, methods, and applications to exercise science. *Exercise and Sport Sciences Reviews, 17*, 423-473.

Fletcher, G.F., Balady, G., Blair, S.N., Blumenthal, J., Caspersen, C., Chaitman, B., Epstein, S., et al. (1992). *American Heart Association position statement on exercise*. American Heart Association.

Haskell, W.L., Lee, I.M., Pate, R.R., Powell, K.E., Blair, S.N., Franklin, B.A., et al. (2007). Physical activity and public health: Updated recommendation for adults from the American College of Sports Medicine and the American Heart Association. *Medicine and Science in Sports and Exercise, 39*(8), 1423-1434.

King, A.C., Haskell, W.L., Taylor, C.B., Kraemer, H.C., & DeBusk, R.F. (1991). Group- vs. home-based exercise training in healthy older men and women. *Journal of the American Medical Association, 266*(11), 1535-1542.

Marcus, B.H., Lewis, B.A., Williams, D.M., Dunsiger, S.I., Jakicic, J.M., Whiteley, J.A., Albrecht, A.E., Napolitano, M.A., Bock, B.C., Tate, D.F., Sciamanna, C.A., & Parisi, A.F. (2007). A comparison of Internet and print-based physical activity interventions. *Archives of Internal Medicine, 167*(9), 944-949.

Marcus, B.H., Napolitano, M.A., Lewis, B.A., King, A.C., Whiteley, J.A., Albrecht, A.E., Parisi, A.F., Pinto, B.M., Bock, B.C., Sciamanna, C.A., Jakicic, J.M., & Papandonatos, G.D. (2007). Examination of print and telephone channels for physical activity promotion: Rationale, design, and baseline data from project STRIDE. *Contemporary Clinical Trials, 28*(1), 90-104.

Marcus, B.H., Nigg, C.R., Riebe, D., & Forsyth, L.H. (2000). Interactive communication strategies: Implications for population-based physical activity promotion. *American Journal of Preventive Medicine, 19*(2), 121-126.

NIH Consensus Development Panel on Physical Activity and Cardiovascular Health. (1996). Physical activity and cardiovascular health. *Journal of the American Medical Association, 276*(3), 241-246.

Pate, R.R., Pratt, M., Blair, S.N., Haskell, W.L., Macera, C.A., Bouchard, C., et al. (1995). Physical activity and public health: A recommendation from the Centers for Disease Control and Prevention and the American College of Sports Medicine. *Journal of the American Medical Association, 273*(5), 402-407.

Prochaska, J.O., & DiClemente, C.C. (1983). The stages and processes of self-change in smoking: Towards an integrative model of change. *Journal of Consulting and Clinical Psychology, 51*(3), 390-395.

U.S. Department of Health and Human Services. (1996). *Physical activity and health: A report of the Surgeon General*. Centers for Disease Control and Prevention, National Center for Chronic Disease Prevention and Health Promotion.

U.S. Department of Health and Human Services. (2000). *Healthy People 2010*. (2nd ed., With Understanding and Improving Health and Objectives for Improving Health. 2 vols.). U.S. Government Printing Office.

U.S. Department of Health and Human Services. *Physical Activity Guidelines for Americans, 2nd edition*. Washington, DC: U.S. Department of Health and Human Services; 2018.

Robert Ross, Jean-Philippe Chaput, Lora M. Giangregorio, Ian Janssen, Travis J. Saunders, Michelle E. Kho, Veronica J. Poitras, Jennifer R. Tomasone, Rasha El-Kotob, Emily C. McLaughlin, Mary Duggan, Julie Carrier, Valerie Carson, Sebastien F. Chastin, Amy E. Latimer-Cheung, Tala Chulak-Bozzer, Guy Faulkner, Stephanie M. Flood, Mary Kate Gazendam, Genevieve N. Healy, Peter T. Katzmarzyk, William Kennedy, Kirstin N. Lane, Amanda Lorbergs, Kaleigh Maclaren, Sharon Marr, Kenneth E. Powell, Ryan E. Rhodes, Amanda Ross-White, Frank Welsh, Juana Willumsen, and Mark S. Tremblay. 2020. Canadian 24-Hour Movement Guidelines for Adults aged 18–64 years and Adults aged 65 years or older: an integration of physical activity, sedentary behaviour, and sleep. *Applied Physiology, Nutrition, and Metabolism*. 45(10 (Suppl. 2)): S57-S102. https://doi.org/10.1139/apnm-2020-0467

Matthews CE, Chen KY, Freedson PS, Buchowski MS, Beech BM, Pate RR, et al. Amount of time spent in sedentary behaviors in the United States, 2003–2004. *Am J Epidemiol* 2008;167:875–81.

Katzmarzyk PT, Powell KE, Jakicic JM, Troiano RP, Piercy K, Tennant B; 2018 PHYSICAL ACTIVITY GUIDELINES ADVISORY COMMITTEE*. Sedentary Behavior and Health: Update from the 2018 Physical Activity Guidelines Advisory Committee. Med Sci Sports Exerc. 2019 Jun;51(6):1227-1241. doi: 10.1249/MSS.0000000000001935. PMID: 31095080; PMCID: PMC6527341.

Marcus BH, Dunsiger S, Pekmezi D, Benitez T, Larsen B, Meyer D. Physical activity outcomes from a randomized trial of a theory- and technology-enhanced intervention for Latinas: the Seamos Activas II study. J Behav Med. 2022 Feb;45(1):1-13. doi: 10.1007/s10865-021-00246-6. Epub 2021 Aug 11. PMID: 34379236.

Mendoza-Vasconez AS, Benitez T, Dunsiger S, Gans KM, Hartman SJ, Linke SE, Larsen BA, Pekmezi D, Marcus BH. Pasos Hacia La Salud II: study protocol for a randomized controlled trial of a theory- and technology-enhanced physical activity intervention for Latina women, compared to the original intervention. Trials. 2022 Aug 1;23(1):621. doi: 10.1186/s13063-022-06575-4. PMID: 35915473; PMCID: PMC9341151.

Pekmezi D, Ainsworth C, Holly T, Williams V, Joseph R, Wang K, Rogers LQ, Marcus B, Desmond R, Demark-Wahnefried W. Physical Activity and Related Psychosocial Outcomes From a Pilot Randomized Trial of an Interactive Voice Response System-Supported Intervention in the Deep South. Health Educ Behav. 2018 Dec;45(6):957-966. doi: 10.1177/1090198118775492. Epub 2018 Jun 8. PMID: 29884069; PMCID: PMC7457542.

Arredondo EM, Schneider J, Torres-Ruiz M, Telles V, Thralls Butte K, West M, Maldonado M, Gallagher K, Roesch S, Ayala GX, Baranowski T. Rationale and design of a pilot randomized controlled trial to increase moderate-to-vigorous physical activity in preadolescent Latina girls and their mothers. Contemp Clin Trials Commun. 2023 Apr 20;33:101137. doi: 10.1016/j.conctc.2023.101137. PMID: 37215388; PMCID: PMC10192392.

Paul Jansons, Lauren Robins, Lisa O'Brien, Terry Haines,

Gym-based exercise and home-based exercise with telephone support have similar outcomes when used as maintenance programs in adults with chronic health conditions: a randomised trial, Journal of Physiotherapy, Volume 63, Issue 3, 2017, Pages 154-160, ISSN 1836-9553, https://doi.org/10.1016/j.jphys.2017.05.018.

Chapter 2

Bandura, A. (1977). Self-efficacy: Toward a unifying theory of behavior change. *Psychological Reviews, 84*(2), 191-215.

Bandura, A. (1986). *Social foundations of thought and action: A social cognitive theory.* Prentice Hall.

Bandura, A. (1997). *Self-efficacy: The exercise of control.* W.H. Freeman.

Dunn, A.L., Marcus, B.H., Kampert, J.B., Garcia, M.E., Kohl, H.W., III, & Blair, S.N. (1997). Reduction in cardiovascular disease risk factors: 6-month results from Project Active. *Preventive Medicine, 26*(6), 883-892.

Horiuchi, S., Tsuda, A., Kobayashi, H., Fallon, E., & Sakano, Y. (2017). Self-efficacy, pros, and cons as variables associated with adjacent stages of change for regular exercise in Japanese college students. *Journal of Health Psychology, 22*(8). 993-1003. https://doi.org/10.1177/1359105315621779

Janis, I.L., & Mann, L. (1977). *Decision making: A psychological analysis of conflict, choice and commitment.* Free Press.

Marcus, B.H., Bock, B.C., Pinto, B.M., Forsyth, L.H., Roberts, M.B., & Traficante, R.M. (1998). Efficacy of an individualized, motivationally tailored physical activity intervention. *Annals of Behavioral Medicine, 20*(3), 174-180.

Marcus, B.H., Rossi, J.S., Selby, V.C., Niaura, R.S., & Abrams, D.B. (1992). The stages and processes of exercise adoption and maintenance in a worksite sample. *Health Psychology, 11*(6), 386-395.

Marcus, B.H., Selby, V.C., Niaura, R.S., & Rossi, J.S. (1992). Self-efficacy and the stages of exercise behavior change. *Research Quarterly for Exercise and Sport, 63*(1), 60-66.

Marcus, B.H., & Simkin, L.R. (1993). The stages of exercise behavior. *Journal of Sports Medicine and Physical Fitness, 33*(1), 83-88.

Prochaska, J.O. (1979). *Systems of psychotherapy: A transtheoretical analysis.* Dorsey Press.

Prochaska, J.O., & DiClemente, C.C. (1983). The stages and processes of self-change in smoking: Toward an integrative model of change. *Journal of Consulting and Clinical Psychology, 51*(3), 390-395.

Prochaska, J.O., DiClemente, C.C., & Norcross, J.C. (1992). In search of how people change: Applications to addictive behaviors. *American Psychologist, 47*(9), 1102-1114.

Prochaska, J.O., Velicer, W.F., DiClemente, C.C., & Fava, J. (1988). Measuring processes of change: Applications to the cessation of smoking. *Journal of Consulting and Clinical Psychology, 56*(4), 520-528.

Skinner, B.F. (1953). *Science and human behavior.* Free Press.

U.S. Department of Health and Human Services. (2018). *Physical activity and health: A report of the Surgeon General.* Centers for Disease Control and Prevention, National Center for Chronic Disease Prevention and Health Promotion.

Cardinal BJ (1999) Extended stage of change model of physical activity behavior. *Journal of Human Movement Studies* 37: 37–54.

Cardinal BJ, Levy SS (2000) Are sedentary behaviors terminable? *Journal of Human Movement Studies* 38: 137–150.

Fallon EA, Hausenblas HA (2001) Transtheoretical model of behavior change: Does the termination stage exist for exercise. *Journal of Human Movement Studies* 40: 465–479.

Fallon EA, Hausenblas HA (2004) Transtheoretical model: In termination applicable to exercise? *American Journal of Health Studies* 35: 44.

Fallon EA, Hausenblas HA, Nigg CR (2005) The transtheoretical model and exercise adherence: Examining construct associations in later stages of change. *Psychology of Sport and Exercise* 6: 629–641.

Horiuchi S, Tsuda A, Watanabe Y, Fukamachi S, Samejima S. Validity of the six stages of change for exercise. *Journal of Health Psychology.* 2013;18(4):518-527. doi:10.1177/1359105312437262

Chapter 3

Adams, M.A., Hurley, J.C., Todd, M., Bhuiyan, N., Jarrett, C.L., Tucker, W.J., Hollingshead, K.E., & Angadi, S.S. (2017). Adaptive goal setting and financial incentives: A 2 × 2 factorial randomized controlled trial to increase adults' physical activity. *BMC Public Health, 17*(1), 286. https://doi.org/10.1186/s12889-017-4197-8

Badland, H., & Schofield, G. (2005). Transport, urban design, and physical activity: An evidence-based update. *Transport Research Part D: Transport and Environment, 10*(3), 177-196.

Bandura, A. (1986). *Social foundations of thought and action: A social cognitive theory.* Prentice Hall.

Bandura, A. (1997). *Self-efficacy: The exercise of control.* W.H. Freeman and Co.

Bandura, A. (2001). Social cognitive theory: An agentic perspective. *Annual Review of Psychology, 52*, 1-26.

Epstein, L.H. (1998). Integrating theoretical approaches to promote physical activity. *American Journal of Preventive Medicine, 15*(4), 257-265.

Glanz, K., & Rimer, B.K. (1995). *Theory at a glance: A guide for health promotion practice.* U.S. Department of Health and Human Services, Public Health Service, National Institutes of Health, and National Cancer Institute.

Humpel, N., Owen, N., & Leslie, E. (2002). Environmental factors associated with adults' participation in physical activity. *American Journal of Preventive Medicine, 22*(3), 188-199.

Ismail, N.A., Hashim, H.A., & Yusof, H.A. (2022). Physical activity and exergames among older adults: A scoping review. (2022). *Games for Health Journal, 11*(1), 1-17. https://doi.org/10.1089/g4h.2021.0104

Janis, I.L., & Mann, L. (1977). *Decision making: A psychological analysis of conflict, choice, and commitment.* Collier Macmillan.

Lewis, B.A., Marcus, B.H., Pate, R.P., & Dunn, A.L. (2002). Psychosocial mediators of physical activity behavior among adults and children. *American Journal of Preventive Medicine, 23*(2S), 26-35.

Marcus, B.H., Rakowski, W., & Rossi, J.S. (1992). Assessing motivational readiness and decision-making for exercise. *Health Psychology, 11*(4), 257-261.

Marcus, B.H., Selby, V.C., Niaura, R.S., & Rossi, J.S. (1992). Self-efficacy and the stages of exercise behavior change. *Research Quarterly for Exercise and Sport, 63*(1), 60-66.

Marlatt, G.A., & Gordon, J.R. (1985). *Relapse prevention: Maintenance strategies in the treatment of addictive behaviors.* Guilford Press.

McLeroy, K.R., Bibeau, D., Steckler, A., & Glanz, K. (1988). An ecological perspective on health promotion programs. *Health Education Quarterly, 15*(4), 351-377.

Mendoza-Vasconez, A.S., Arredondo, E.M., Larsen, B., et al. (2021). Lapse, relapse, and recovery in physical activity interventions for Latinas: A survival analysis. *International Journal of Behavioral Medicine, 28,* 540-551. https://doi.org/10.1007/s12529-020-09943-z.

Paffenbarger, R.S., Hyde, R.T., Wing, A.L., & Hsieh, C. (1986). Physical activity, all-cause mortality, and longevity of college alumni. *New England Journal of Medicine, 314*(10, 605-613.

Sallis, J.F., Bauman, A., & Pratt, M. (1998). Environmental and policy interventions to promote physical activity. *American Journal of Preventive Medicine, 15*(4), 379-397.

Sallis, J.F., Hovell, L.M.R., Hofstetter, C.R., Faucher, P., Elder, J.P., Blanchard, J., et al. (1989). A multivariate study of determinants of vigorous exercise in a community sample. *Preventive Medicine, 18*(1), 20-34.

Skinner, B.F. (1953). *Science and human behavior.* Free Press.

Street, T.D., Lacey, S.J., & Langdon, R.R. (2017). Gaming your way to health: A systematic review of exergaming programs to increase health and exercise behaviors in adults. *Games for Health Journal, 6*(3), 136-146. https://doi.org/10.1089/g4h.2016.0102

U.S. Department of Health and Human Services. (1996). *Physical activity and health: A report of the Surgeon General.* Centers for Disease Control and Prevention, National Center for Chronic Disease Prevention and Health Promotion.

Wankel, L.M. (1984). Decision-making and social support strategies for increasing exercise involvement. *Journal of Cardiac Rehabilitation, 4,* 124-135.

Sallis JF. Needs and Challenges Related to Multilevel Interventions: Physical Activity Examples. *Health Education & Behavior.* 2018;45(5):661-667. doi:10.1177/1090198118796458

Salvo G, Lashewicz BM, Doyle-Baker PK, McCormack GR. Neighbourhood Built Environment Influences on Physical Activity among Adults: A Systematized Review of Qualitative Evidence. *International Journal of Environmental Research and Public Health.* 2018; 15(5):897. https://doi.org/10.3390/ijerph15050897

Israel, Barbara A.; Schulz, Amy J.; Parker, Edith A.; Becker, Adam B. (1998). "REVIEW OF COMMUNITY-BASED RESEARCH: Assessing Partnership Approaches to Improve Public Health". *Annual Review of Public Health.* **19**: 173–202. doi:10.1146/annurev.publhealth.19.1.173. PMID 9611617.

Rogers, Everett (16 August 2003). *Diffusion of Innovations, 5th Edition.* Simon and Schuster. ISBN 978-0-7432-5823-4.

Larsen, B., Dunsiger, S.I., Pekmezi, D., Linke, S., Hartman, S.J., & Marcus, B.H. (2021). Psychosocial mediators of physical activity change in a web-based intervention for Latinas. *Health Psychology, 40*(1), 21-29. https://doi.org/10.1037/hea0001041

Chapter 4

Abbaspour, S., Farmanbar, R., Njafi, F., Ghiasvand, A.M., & Dehghankar, L. (2017). Decisional balance and self-efficacy of physical activity among the elderly in Rasht in 2013 based on the transtheoretical model. *Electronic Physician, 9*(5), 4447-4453. https://doi.org/10.19082/4447

Baird, J.F., Silveira, S.L., & Motl, R.W. (2021). Social cognitive theory and physical activity in older adults with multiple sclerosis. *International Journal of MS Care, 23*(1), 21-25. https://doi.org/10.7224/1537-2073.2019-071

Bandura, A. (1986). *Social foundations of thought and action: A social cognitive theory.* Prentice Hall.

Bandura, A. (1997). *Self-efficacy: The exercise of control.* W.H. Freeman.

Baranowski, T., Anderson, C., & Carmack, C. (1998). Mediating variable framework in physical activity interventions: How are we doing? How might we do better? *American Journal of Preventive Medicine, 15*(4), 266-297.

Baron, R.M., & Kenny, D.A. (1986). The moderator–mediator variable distinction in social psychological research: Conceptual, strategic, and statistical considerations. *Journal of Personality and Social Psychology, 51*(6), 1173-1182.

Bauman, A.E., Sallis, J.F., Dzewaltowski, D.A., & Owen, N. (2002). Toward a better understanding of the influences on physical activity: The role of determinants, correlates, causal variables, mediators, moderators, and confounders. *American Journal of Preventive Medicine, 23*(2S), 5-14.

Bernard, P., Romain, A.J., Trouillet, R., et al. (2014). Validation of the TTM processes of change measure for physical activity in an adult French sample. *International Journal of Behavioral Medicine, 21*, 402–410. https://doi.org/10.1007/s12529-013-9292-3

Bradley, J.M., Wilson, J.J., Hayes, K., Kent, L., McDonough, S., Tully, M.A., Bradbury, I., Kirk, A., Cosgrove, D., Convery, R., et al. (2015). Sedentary behaviour and physical activity in bronchiectasis: A cross-sectional study. *BMC Pulmonary Medicine, 15*, 61. https://doi.org/10.1186/s12890-015-0046-7

Brassington, G.S., Atienza, A.A., Perczek, R.E., DiLorenzo, T.M., & King, A.C. (2002). Intervention-related cognitive versus social mediators of exercise adherence in the elderly. *American Journal of Preventive Medicine, 23*(2S), 80-86.

Cardinal, B.J., Tuominen, K.J., & Rintala, P. (2003). Psychometric assessment of Finnish versions of exercise-related measures of transtheoretical model constructs. *International Journal of Behavioral Medicine, 10*(1), 31-43.

Chu, S.F., & Wang, H.H. (2022). Outcome expectations and older adults with knee osteoarthritis: Their exercise outcome expectations in relation to perceived health, self-efficacy, and fear of falling. *Healthcare, 11*(1), 57. https://doi.org/10.3390/healthcare11010057

Cohen, S., Mermelstein, R., Kamarck, T., & Hoberman, H.M. (1985). Measuring the functional components of social support. In I.G. Sarason & B.R. Sarason (Eds.), *Social support: Theory, research, and applications* (pp. 73-94). Martinus Nijhoff.

Courneya, K.S., & McAuley, E. (1995). Cognitive mediators of the social influence–exercise adherence relationship: A test of the theory of planned behavior. *Journal of Behavioral Medicine, 18*(5), 499-515.

Crozier, A.J. & Spink, K.S. (2017). Effect of manipulating descriptive norms and positive outcome expectations on physical activity of university students during exams. *Health Communication, 32*(6), 784-790. https://doi.org/10.1080/10410236.2016.1172295

DiClemente, C.C., Prochaska, J.O., Fairhurst, S.K., Velicer, W.F., Rossi, J.J., & Velasquez, M. (1991). The process of smoking cessation: An analysis of precontemplation, contemplation, and preparation stages of change. *Journal of Consulting and Clinical Psychology, 59*(2), 295-304.

Dishman, R., Jackson, A.S., & Bray, M.S. (2010). Validity of processes of change in physical activity among college students in the TIGER Study. *Annals of Behavioral Medicine, 40*, 164-175.

Dishman, R.K., Motl, R.W., Saunders, R., Felton, G., Ward, D.S., Dowda, M., & Pate, R.R. (2005). Enjoyment mediates effects of a school-based physical activity intervention. *Medicine and Science in Sports and Exercise, 37*(3), 478-487.

Dunn, A.L., Marcus, B.H., Kampert, J.B., Garcia, M.E., Kohl, H.W., & Blair, S.N. (1997). Reduction in cardiovascular disease risk factors: 6-month results from Project Active. *Preventive Medicine, 26*(6), 883-892.

Fjeldsoe, B.S., Miller, Y.D., & Marshall, A.L. (2013). Social cognitive mediators of the effect of the MobileMums intervention on physical activity. *Health Psychology, 32*(7), 729-738. https://doi.org/10.1037/a0027548

Frerichs, L., Bess, K., Young, T.L., et al. (2020). A cluster randomized trial of a community-based intervention among African-American adults: Effects on dietary and physical activity outcomes. *Prevention Science, 21*, 344-354. https://doi.org/10.1007/s11121-019-01067-5

Hallam, J., & Petosa, R. (1998). A worksite intervention to enhance social cognitive theory constructs to promote exercise adherence. *American Journal of Health Promotion, 13*(1), 4-7.

Harada, K. (2022). Effectiveness, moderators and mediators of self-regulation intervention on older adults' exercise behavior: A randomized, controlled crossover trial. *International Journal of Behavioral Medicine, 29*, 659-675. https://doi.org/10.1007/s12529-021-10049-3

Hartman, S.J., Dunsiger, S.I., Pekmezi, D.W., Barbera, B., Neighbors, C.J., Marquez, B., & Marcus, B.H. (2011). Impact of baseline BMI upon the success of Latina participants enrolled in a 6-month physical activity intervention. *Journal of Obesity*, 921916. https://doi.org/10.1155/2011/921916

Howlett, N., Trivedi, D., Troop, N.A., & Chater, A.M. (2019). Are physical activity interventions for healthy inactive adults effective in promoting behaviour change and maintenance, and which behaviour change techniques are effective? A systematic review and meta-analysis. *Translational Behavioral Medicine, 9*, 147-157.

Janis, I.L., & Mann, L. (1977). *Decision making: A psychological analysis of conflict, choice, and commitment.* Collier Macmillan.

Jiménez-Zazo, F., Romero-Blanco, C., Castro-Lemus, N., Dorado-Suárez, A., & Aznar, S. (2020). Transtheoretical model for physical activity in older adults: Systematic review. *International Journal of Environmental Research and Public Health, 17*(24), 9262. https://doi.org/10.3390/ijerph17249262

Kanning, M. (2010). Physically active patients with coronary artery disease: A longitudinal investigation of the processes of exercise behaviour change. *British Journal of Health Psychology, 15*(3), 583-597. https://doi.org/10.1348/135910709X477476

Kendzierski, D., & DeCarlo, K.J. (1991). Physical activity enjoyment scale: Two validation studies. *Journal of Sport and Exercise Psychology, 13*(1), 50-64.

King, A.C., Stokols, D., Talin, B., Brassington, G.S., & Killingsworth, R. (2002). Theoretical approaches to the promotion of physical activity: Forging a transdisciplinary paradigm. *American Journal of Preventive Medicine, 23*(2S), 15-25.

Koring, M., Richert, J., Parschau, L., Ernsting, A., Lippke, S., & Schwarzer, R. (2012). A combined planning and self-efficacy intervention to promote physical activity: A multiple mediation analysis. *Psychology, Health & Medicine, 17*(4), 488-498. https://doi.org/10.1080/13548506.2011.608809

Kouvonen, A., De Vogli, R., Stafford, M., Shipley, M.J., Marmot, M.G., Cox, T., Vahtera, J., Väänänen, A., Heponiemi, T., Singh-Manoux, A., & Kivimäki, M. (2012). Social support and the likelihood of maintaining and improving levels of physical activity: The Whitehall II Study. *European Journal of Public Health, 22*(4), 514-518. https://doi.org/10.1093/eurpub/ckr091

Larsen, B., Dunsiger, S.I., Pekmezi, D., Linke, S., Hartman, S.J., & Marcus, B.H. (2021). Psychosocial mediators of physical activity change in a web-based intervention for Latinas. *Health Psychology, 40*(1), 21-29. https://doi.org/10.1037/hea0001041

Leslie, E., Owen, N., Salmon, J., Bauman, A., Sallis, J.F., & Kai Lo, S. (1999). Insufficiently active Australian college students: Perceived personal, social, and environmental influences. *Preventive Medicine, 28*(1), 20-27.

Lewis, B.A., Forsyth, L.H., Pinto, B.M., Bock, B.C., Roberts, M., & Marcus, B.H. (2006). Psychosocial mediators of physical activity in a randomized controlled intervention trial. *Journal of Sport and Exercise Psychology, 28*, 193-204.

Lewis, B.A., Marcus, B.H., Pate, R.R., & Dunn, A.L. (2002). Psychosocial mediators of physical activity behavior among adults and children. *American Journal of Preventive Medicine, 23*(2S), 26-35.

Lewis, B.A., Williams, D.M., Frayeh, A., & Marcus, B.H. (2016). Self-efficacy versus perceived enjoyment as predictors of physical activity behaviour. *Psychology & Health, 31*(4), 456-469. https://doi.org/10.1080/08870446.2015.1111372

Linke, S., Robinson, C., & Pekmezi, D. (2014). Applying psychological theories to promote healthy lifestyles. *American Journal of Lifestyle Medicine, 8*(1), 4-14.

Marcus, B.H., Bock, B.C., Pinto, B.M., Forsyth, L.H., Roberts, M., & Traficante, R. (1998). Efficacy of individualized, motivationally tailored physical activity intervention. *Annals of Behavioral Medicine, 20*(3), 174-180.

Marcus, B.H., Dunsiger, S.I., Pekmezi, D.W., Larsen, B.A., Bock, B.C., Gans, K.M., Marquez, B., Morrow, K.M., & Tilkemeier, P. (2013). The Seamos Saludables study: A randomized controlled physical activity trial of Latinas. *American Journal of Preventive Medicine, 45*(5), 598-605. https://doi.org/10.1016/j.amepre.2013.07.006

Marcus, B.H., Eaton, C.A., Rossi, J.S., & Harlow, L.L. (1994). Self-efficacy, decision-making, and stages of change: An integrative model of physical exercise. *Journal of Applied Social Psychology, 24*(6), 489-508.

Marcus, B.H., & Owen, N. (1992). Motivational readiness, self-efficacy and decision making for exercise. *Journal of Applied Social Psychology, 22*(1), 3-16.

Marcus, B.H., Rakowski, W., & Rossi, J.S. (1992). Assessing motivational readiness and decision-making for exercise. *Health Psychology, 11*(4), 257-261.

Marcus, B.H., Rossi, J.S., Selby, V.C., Niaura, R.S., & Abrams, D.B. (1992). The stages and processes of exercise adoption and maintenance in a worksite sample. *Health Psychology, 11*(6), 386-395.

Marcus, B.H., Selby, V.C., Niaura, R.S., & Rossi, J.S. (1992). Self-efficacy and the stages of exercise behavior change. *Research Quarterly for Exercise and Sport, 63*(1), 60-66.

Marinac, C.R., Dunsiger, S.I., Marcus, B.H., Rosen, R.K., Gans, K.M., & Hartman, S.J. (2018). Mediators of a physical activity intervention among women with a family history of breast cancer. *Women & Health, 58*(6), 699-713. https://doi.org/10.1080/03630242.2017.1333075

Marquez, B., Dunsiger, S.I., Pekmezi, D., Larsen, B.A., & Marcus, B.H. (2016). Social support and physical activity change in Latinas: Results from the Seamos Saludables trial. *Health Psychology, 35*(12), 1392-1401. https://doi.org/10.1037/hea0000421

McFadden, K., Berry, T., McHugh, T.-L., & Rodgers, W. (2022). Relationships of automatic associations, affect, and outcome expectations with adolescents' impulsive decision to opt into physical activity. *International Journal of Sport and Exercise Psychology, 20*(6), 1734-1751. https://doi.org/10.1080/1612197X.2021.1993961

Mendoza-Vasconez, A.S., Marquez, B., Benitez, T.J., et al. (2018). Psychometrics of the self-efficacy for physical activity scale among a Latina women sample. *BMC Public Health, 18*, 1097. https://doi.org/10.1186/s12889-018-5998-0

Miller, Y.D., Trost, S.G., & Brown, W.J. (2002). Mediators of physical activity behavior change among women with young children. *American Journal of Preventive Medicine, 23*(2S), 98-103.

Miller, Y.D., Trost, S.G., & Brown, W.J. (2006). Will you take care of the kids? Mediating effects of partner support in changing physical activity among women with young children. *American Journal of Preventive Medicine, 23*(2S), 98-103.

Monteiro D., Rodrigues F., & Lopes V. (2021). El apoyo proporcionado por el mejor amigo y la actividad física de alta intensidad en relación con los beneficios y la autoestima global en adolescentes [Social support provided by the best friend and vigorous-intensity physical activity in the relationship between perceived benefits and global self-worth of adolescents]. *Revista de Psicodidáctica, 26*(1), 70-77.

Morrison, J.D., & Stuifbergen, A.K. (2014). Outcome expectations and physical activity in persons with longstanding multiple sclerosis. *Journal of Neuroscience Nursing, 46*(3), 171-179. https://doi.org/10.1097/JNN.0000000000000050

Napolitano, M.A., Papandonatos, G.D., Lewis, B.A., Whiteley, J.A., Williams, D.M., King, A.C., Bock, B.C., Pinto, B., & Marcus, B.H. (2008). Mediators of physical activity behavior change: A multivariate approach. *Health Psychology, 27*(4), 409-418. https://doi.org/10.1037/0278-6133.27.4.409

Nichols, J.F., Willman, E., Caparosa, S., Sallis, J.F., Calfas, K.J., & Rowe, R. (2000). Impact of a worksite behavioral skills intervention. *American Journal of Health Promotion, 14*(4), 218-221.

Oka, R., King, A.C., & Young, D.R. (1995). Sources of social support as predictors of exercise adherence in women and men ages 50 to 65 years. *Women Health Research and Gender Policy, 1*(2), 161-175.

Papandonatos, G.D., Williams, D.M., Jennings, E.G., Napolitano, M.A., Bock, B.C., Dunsiger, S., & Marcus, B.H. (2012). Mediators of physical activity behavior change: Findings from a 12-month randomized controlled trial. *Health Psychology, 31*(4), 512-520. https://doi.org/10.1037/a0026667

Pinto, B.M., Lynn, H., Marcus, B.H., DePue, J., & Goldstein, M.G. (2001). Physician-based activity counseling: Intervention effects on mediators of motivational readiness for exercise. *Annals of Behavioral Medicine, 23*(1), 2-10.

Prochaska, J.O., & DiClemente, C.C. (1983). Stages and processes of self-change of smoking: Toward an integrative model of change. *Journal of Consulting and Clinical Psychology, 51*(3), 390-395.

Resnick, B., Zimmerman, S.I., Orwig, D., Furstenberg, A., & Magaziner, J. (2000). Outcome expectations for exercise scale: Utility and psychometrics. *Journal of Gerontology: Series B: Psychological Sciences and Social Sciences, 55*(6), S352-S356.

Rhodes, R.E., Boudreau, P., Weman Josefsson, K., & Ivarsson, A. (2021) Mediators of physical activity behaviour change interventions among adults: A systematic review and meta-analysis. *Health Psychology Review, 15*(2), 272-286. https://doi.org/10.1080/17437199.2019.1706614

Rhodes, R.E., Janssen, I., Bredin, S.S.D., Warburton, D.E.R., & Bauman, A. (2017). Physical activity: Health impact, prevalence, correlates and interventions. *Psychology & Health, 32*(8), 942-975. https://doi.org/10.1080/08870446.2017.1325486

Rhodes, R.E., & Pfaeffli, L.A. (2010). Mediators of physical activity behaviour change among adult non-clinical populations: A review update. *International Journal of Behavioral Nutrition and Physical Activity, 7*, 37. https://doi.org/10.1186/1479-5868-7-37

Rodrigues, F., Monteiro, D., & Lopes, V.P. (2023). The mediation role of perceived benefits and barriers in the relationship between support provided by significant others and physical activity of adolescents. *Perceptual and Motor Skills, 130*(2), 902-922. https://doi.org/10.1177/00315125231151780

Rosen, C.S. (2000). Is the sequencing of change processes by stage consistent across health problems? A meta-analysis. *Health Psychology, 19*(6), 593-604.

Rovniak, L.S., Anderson, E.S., Winett, R.A., & Stephens, R.S. (2002). Social cognitive determinants of physical activity in young adults: A prospective structural equation analysis. *Annals of Behavioral Medicine, 24*(2), 149-156.

Sallis, J.F., Calfas, K.J., Alcaraz, J.E., Gehrman, C., & Johnson, M.F. (1999). Potential mediators of change in a physical activity promotion course for university students: Project GRAD. *Annals of Behavioral Medicine, 21*, 149-158,

Sallis, J.F., Grossman, R.M., Pinski, R.B., Patterson, T.L., & Nader, P.R. (1987). The development of scales to measure social support for diet and exercise behaviors. *Preventive Medicine, 16*(6), 825-836.

Sallis, J.F., Pinski, R.B., Grossman, R.M., Patterson, T.L., & Nader, P.R. (1988). The development of self-efficacy scales for health-related diet and exercise behaviors. *Health Education Research, 3*(3), 283-292.

Sarason, I.G., & Sarason, B.R. (1985). *Social support: Theory, research, and applications.* Martinus Nijhoff.

Stevens, M., Lemmink, K.A., de Greef, M.H., & Rispens, P. (2000). Gronigen Active Living Model (GALM): Stimulating physical activity in sedentary older adults; first results. *Preventive Medicine, 31*(5), 547-553.

Stoddard, A.M., Palombo, R., Troped, P.J., Sorensen, G. & Will, J.C. (2004). Cardiovascular disease risk reduction: The Massachusetts WISEWOMAN project. *Journal of Women's Health* (Larchmont), *13*(5), 539-546.

Taymoori, P., & Revalds Lubans, D. (2008). Mediators of behavior change in two tailored physical activity interventions for adolescent girls. *Psychology of Sport and Exercise, 9*(5), 605-619.

U.S. Department of Health and Human Services. (1996). *Physical activity and health: A report of the Surgeon General.* Centers for Disease Control and Prevention, National Center for Chronic Disease Prevention and Health Promotion.

Wankel, L.M. (1993). The importance of enjoyment to adherence and psychological benefits from physical activity. *International Journal of Sport Psychology, 24*(2), 151-169.

Williams, D.M., Anderson, E.S., & Winett, R.A. (2005). A review of the outcome expectancy construct in physical activity research. *Annals of Behavioral Medicine, 29*(1), 70-79.

Williams, D.M., Papandonatos, G.D., Napolitano, M.A., & Lewis, B.A. (2006). Perceived enjoyment moderates the efficacy of an individually tailored physical activity intervention. *Journal of Sports and Exercise Psychology, 28*(3), 300-309.

Yang, C.-H., Maher, J.P., & Conroy, D.E. (2015). Implementation of behavior change techniques in mobile applications for physical activity. *American Journal of Preventive Medicine, 48*(4), 452-455.

Teixeira PJ, Carraça EV, Marques MM, Rutter H, Oppert JM, De Bourdeaudhuij I, Lakerveld J, Brug J. Successful behavior change in obesity interventions in adults: a systematic review of self-regulation mediators. BMC Med. 2015 Apr 16;13:84. doi: 10.1186/s12916-015-0323-6. PMID: 25907778; PMCID: PMC4408562.

Lindsay Smith, G., Banting, L., Eime, R. et al. The association between social support and physical activity in older adults: a systematic review. *Int J Behav Nutr Phys Act* **14**, 56 (2017). https://doi.org/10.1186/s12966-017-0509-8

Mendonça G, Cheng LA, Mélo EN, de Farias Júnior JC. Physical activity and social support in adolescents: a systematic review. Health Educ Res. 2014 Oct;29(5):822-39. doi: 10.1093/her/cyu017. Epub 2014 May 8. PMID: 24812148.

Pekmezi DW, Neighbors CJ, Lee CS, Gans KM, Bock BC, Morrow KM, Marquez B, Dunsiger S, Marcus BH. A culturally adapted physical activity intervention for Latinas: a randomized controlled trial. Am J Prev Med. 2009 Dec;37(6):495-500. doi: 10.1016/j.amepre.2009.08.023. PMID: 19944914; PMCID: PMC2814545.

Klompstra L, Deka P, Almenar L, et al. Physical activity enjoyment, exercise motivation, and physical activity in patients with heart failure: A mediation analysis. *Clinical Rehabilitation.* 2022;36(10):1324-1331. doi:10.1177/02692155221103696

Chapter 5

American Heart Association. (1984a). *Dancing for a healthy heart.*

American Heart Association. (1984b). *Running for a healthy heart.*

American Heart Association. (1984c). *Swimming for a healthy heart.*

American Heart Association. (1984d). *Walking for a healthy heart.*

American Heart Association. (1989). *Cycling for a healthy heart.*

Barnes, P.M., & Schoenborn, C.A. (2003). *Physical activity among adults: United States, 2000.* Advance data from vital and health statistics; no. 333. Hyattsville, MD: National Center for Health Statistics.

Benitez, T.J., Dunsiger, S., Marquez, B., Larsen, B., Pekmezi, D., & Marcus, B.H. (2022). Increases in muscle-strengthening activities among Latinas in Seamos Saludables. *Health Education & Behavior, 49*(3), 446-454. https://doi.org/10.1177/

Bennie, J.A., De Cocker, K., Teychenne, M.J., Brown, W.J., & Biddle, S.J.H. (2019). The epidemiology of aerobic physical activity and muscle-strengthening activity guideline adherence among 383,928 U.S. adults. Int J Behav Nutr Phys Act, 16(1), 34. https://doi.org/10.1186/s12966-019-0797-2

Bennie, J.A., Teychenne, M.J., De Cocker, K., & Biddle, S.J. (2019). Associations between aerobic and muscle-strengthening exercise with depressive symptom severity among 17,839 US adults. Preventive medicine, 121, 121-127.

Bock, B.C., Marcus, B.H., Pinto, B., & Forsyth, L. (2001). Maintenance of physical activity following an individualized motivationally tailored intervention. *Annals of Behavioral Medicine, 23*(2), 79-87.

Centers for Disease Control and Prevention. (2022, February 17). Adult physical inactivity prevalence maps by race/ethnicity. www.cdc.gov/physicalactivity/data/inactivity-prevalence-maps/index.html

Dishman, R.K. (1994). *Advances in exercise adherence.* Human Kinetics.

Dunn, A.L., Marcus, B.H., Kampert, J.B., Garcia, M.E., Kohl, H.W., III, & Blair, S.N. (1999). Comparison of lifestyle and structured interventions to increase physical activity and cardio-respiratory fitness: A randomized trial. *Journal of the American Medical Association, 281*(4), 327-334.

Joseph, R.P., Durant, N.H., Benitez, T.J., & Pekmezi, D.W. (2014). Internet-based physical activity interventions. *American Journal of Lifestyle Medicine, 8*(1), 42-68. https://doi.org/10.1177/1559827613498059

Kahlert, D. (2015). Maintenance of physical activity: Do we know what we are talking about? *Preventive Medicine Reports, 2*, 178-180. https://doi.org/10.1016/j.pmedr.2015.02.013

Linke, S.E., Dunsiger, S.I., Gans, K.M., Hartman, S.J., Pekmezi, D., Larsen, B.A., Mendoza-Vasconez, A.S., & Marcus, B.H. (2019). Association between physical activity intervention website use and physical activity levels among Spanish-speaking Latinas: Randomized controlled trial. *Journal of Medical Internet Research, 21*(7), e13063.

Marcus, B.H., Bock, B.C., Pinto, B.M., Forsyth, L.H., Roberts, M.B., & Traficante, R.M. (1998). Efficacy of an individualized, motivationally-tailored physical activity intervention. *Annals of Behavioral Medicine, 20*(3), 174-180.

Marcus, B.H., Dubbert, P.M., Forsyth, L.H., McKenzie, T.L., Stone, E.J., Dunn, A.L., & Blair, S.N. (2000). Physical activity behavior change: Issues in adoption and maintenance. *Health Psychology, 19*(1), 32-41.

Marcus, B.H., Dunsiger, S., Pekmezi, D., Benitez, T., Larsen, B., & Meyer, D. (2022). Physical activity outcomes from a randomized trial of a theory- and technology-enhanced intervention for Latinas: The Seamos Activas II study. *Journal of Behavioral Medicine, 45*, 1-13. https://doi.org/10.1007/s10865-021-00246-6

Marcus, B.H., Dunsiger, S.I., Pekmezi, D.W., Larsen, B.A., Bock, B.C., Gans, K.M., Marquez, B., Morrow, K.M., & Tilkemeier, P. (2013). The Seamos Saludables study: A randomized controlled physical activity trial of Latinas. *American Journal of Preventive Medicine, 45*(5), 598-605. https://doi.org/10.1016/j.amepre.2013.07.006

Marcus, B.H., Emmons, K.M., Simkin-Silverman, L.R., Linnan, L.A., Taylor, E.R., Bock, B.C., et al. (1998). Evaluation of motivationally tailored vs. standard self-help physical activity interventions at the workplace. *American Journal of Health Promotion, 12*(4), 246-253.

Marcus, B.H., Hartman, S.J., Larsen, B.A., Pekmezi, D., Dunsiger, S.I., Linke, S., Marquez, B., Gans, K.M., Bock, B.C., Mendoza-Vasconez, A.S., Noble, M.L., & Rojas, C. (2016). Pasos Hacia la Salud: A randomized controlled trial of an Internet-delivered physical activity intervention for Latinas. *The International Journal of Behavioral Nutrition and Physical Activity, 13*, 62. https://doi.org/10.1186/s12966-016-0385-7

Marcus, B.H., Hartman, S.J., Pekmezi, D., Dunsiger, S.I., Linke, S.E., Marquez, B., Gans, K.M., Bock, B.C., Larsen, B.A., & Rojas, C. (2015). Using interactive Internet technology to promote physical activity in Latinas: Rationale, design, and baseline findings of Pasos Hacia la Salud. *Contemporary Clinical Trials, 44*, 149-158. https://doi.org/10.1016/j.cct.2015.08.004

Marcus, B.H., Larsen, B.A., Linke, S.E., Hartman, S.J., Pekmezi, D., Benitez, T., Sallis, J., Mendoza-Vasconez, A.S., & Dunsiger, S.I. (2021). Long-term physical activity outcomes in the Seamos Activas II trial. *Preventive Medicine Reports, 24*, 101628.

Marcus, B.H., Lewis, B.A., Williams, D.M., Whiteley, J. A., Albrecht, A.E., Jakicic, J.M., Parisi, A.F., Hogan, J.W., Napolitano, M.A., & Bock, B.C. (2007). Step Into Motion: A randomized trial examining the relative efficacy of Internet vs. print-based physical activity interventions. *Contemporary Clinical Trials, 28*(6), 737-747.

Marcus, B.H., Napolitano, M.A., King, A.C., Lewis, B.A., Whiteley, J.A., Albrecht, A.E., Parisi, A.F., Bock, B.C., Pinto, B.M., Sciamanna, C., Jakicic, J.M., & Papandonatos, G.D. (2007). Telephone versus print delivery of an individualized motivationally tailored physical activity intervention: Project STRIDE. *Health Psychology, 26*(4), 401-409.

Marcus, B.H., Napolitano, M.A., Lewis, B.A., King, A.C., Whiteley, J.A., Albrecht, A.E., Parisi, A.F., Pinto, B.M., Bock, B.C., Sciamanna, C.A., Jakicic, J.M., & Papandonatos, G.D. (2007). Examination of print and telephone channels for physical activity promotion: Rationale, design, and baseline data from project STRIDE. *Contemporary Clinical Trials, 28*(1), 90-104.

McEwan, D., Rhodes, R.E., & Beauchamp, M. (2022). What happens when the party is over? Sustaining physical activity behaviors after intervention cessation. *Behavioral Medicine*, 1-9. https://doi.org/10.1080/08964289.2020.1750335

Pekmezi, D., Ainsworth, C., Desmond, R., Pisu, M., Williams, V., Wang, K., Holly, T., Meneses, K., Bess Marcus, B., & Demark-Wahnefried, W. (2020). Physical activity maintenance following home-based, individually tailored print interventions for African American women. *Health Promotion Practice, 21*(2), 268-276. https://doi.org/10.1177/1524839918798819

Pekmezi, D., Ainsworth, C., Joseph, R., Bray, M.S., Kvale, E., Isaac, S., Desmond, R., Meneses, K., Marcus, B., & Demark-Wahnefried, W. (2016). Rationale, design, and baseline findings from HIPP: A randomized controlled trial testing a home-based, individually-tailored physical activity print intervention for African American women in the Deep South. *Contemporary Clinical Trials, 47*, 340-348.

Pekmezi, D., Ainsworth, C., Joseph, R.P., Williams, V., Desmond, R., Meneses, K., Marcus, B., Demark-Wahnefried, W. (2017). Pilot trial of a home-based physical activity program for African American women. *Medicine & Science in Sports & Exercise, 49*(12), 2528-2536. https://doi.org/10.1249/MSS.0000000000001370

Pekmezi, D., Dunsiger, S., Gans, K., Bock, B., Gaskins, R., Marquez, B., ,Christina Lee, C., Neighbors, C., Jennings, E., Tilkemeier, P., & Marcus, B. (2012). Rationale, design, and baseline findings from Seamos Saludables: A randomized controlled trial testing the efficacy of a culturally and linguistically adapted, computer- tailored physical activity intervention for Latinas. *Contemporary Clinical Trials, 33*(6), 1261-1271. https://doi.org/10.1016/j.cct.2012.07.005

Pekmezi, D.W., Neighbors, C.J., Lee, C.S., Gans, K.M., Bock, B.C., Morrow, K.M., Marquez, B., Dunsiger, S., & Marcus, B.H. (2009). A culturally adapted physical activity intervention for Latinas: A randomized controlled trial. *American Journal of Preventive Medicine, 37*(6), 495-500. https://doi.org/10.1016/j.amepre.2009.08.023

Pew Research Center. (2021, April 7). Internet/broadband fact sheet. www.pewresearch.org/internet/fact-sheet/internet-broadband/

van den Berg, M., Schoones, J., & Vliet Vlieland, T. (2007). Internet-based physical activity interventions: A systematic review of the literature. *Journal of Medical Internet Research, 9*(3), e26. https://doi.org/10.2196/jmir.9.3.e26

Momma H, Kawakami R, Honda T, Sawada SS. Muscle-strengthening activities are associated with lower risk and mortality in major non-communicable diseases: a systematic review and meta-analysis of cohort studies. Br J Sports Med. 2022 Jul;56(13):755-763. doi: 10.1136/bjsports-2021-105061. Epub 2022 Feb 28. PMID: 35228201; PMCID: PMC9209691.

Bennie JA, Shakespear-Druery J, De Cocker K. Muscle-strengthening exercise epidemiology: a new frontier in chronic disease prevention. *Sports Medicine-Open.* 2020; **6**: 1–8.

Chapter 6

Ainsworth, M.C., Pekmezi, D., Bowles, H., Ehlers, D., McAuley, E., Courneya, K.S., & Rogers, L.Q. (2018). Acceptability of a mobile phone app for measuring time use in breast cancer survivors (Life in a Day): Mixed-methods study. *JMIR Cancer, 4*(1), e9. https://doi.org/10.2196/cancer.8951

Bassett, D.R. Jr., Wyatt, H.R., Thompson, H., Peters, J.C., & Hill, J.O. (2010). Pedometer-measured physical activity and health behaviors in U.S. adults. *Medicine & Science in Sports & Exercise, 42*(10), 1819-1825. https://doi.org/10.1249/MSS.0b013e3181dc2e54

Borg, G. (1998). *Perceived exertion and pain scales.* Human Kinetics.

Dooley, E.E., Golaszewski, N.M., & Bartholomew, J.B. (2017). Estimating accuracy at exercise intensities: A comparative study of self-monitoring heart rate and physical activity wearable devices. *JMIR mHealth uhHalth, 5*(3), e34. https://doi.org/10.2196/mhealth.7043

Dowd, K.P., Szeklicki, R., Minetto, M.A., Murphy, M.H., Polito, A., Ghigo, E., van der Ploeg, H., Ekelund, U., Maciaszek, J., Stemplewski, R., Tomczak, M., & Donnelly, A.E. (2018). A systematic literature review of reviews on techniques for physical activity measurement in adults: A DEDIPAC study. *International Journal of Behavioral Nutrition and Physical Activity 15*, 15. https://doi.org/10.1186/s12966-017-0636-2

Falter, M., Budts, W., Goetschalckx, K., Cornelissen, V., & Buys, R. (2019). Accuracy of Apple Watch measurements for heart rate and energy expenditure in patients with cardiovascular disease: Cross-sectional study. *JMIR mHealth uHealth, 7*(3), e11889. https://doi.org/10.2196/11889

Germini, F., Noronha, N., Borg Debono, V., Abraham Philip, B., Pete, D., Navarro, T., Keepanasseril, A., Parpia, S., de Wit, K., & Iorio, A. (2022). Accuracy and acceptability of wrist-wearable activity-tracking devices: Systematic review of the literature. *Journal of Medical Internet Research, 24*(1), e30791. https://doi.org/10.2196/30791

Heyward, V.H. (2006). *Advanced fitness assessment and exercise prescription* (5th ed.). Human Kinetics.

Hoenemeyer, T.W., Cole, W.W., Oster, R.A., Pekmezi, D.W., Pye, A., & Demark-Wahnefried, W. (2022). Test/retest reliability and validity of remote vs. in-person anthropometric and physical performance assessments in cancer survivors and supportive partners. *Cancers, 14*(4), 1075. https://doi.org/10.3390/cancers14041075

Lee, I., Shiroma E.J., Kamada, M., Bassett, D.R., Matthews, CE, & Buring, J.E. (2019). Association of step volume and intensity with all-cause mortality in older women. *JAMA Internal Medicine, 179*(8), 1105-1112. https://doi.org/10.1001/jamainternmed.2019.0899

Marcus, B.H., & Simkin, L.R. (1993). The stages of exercise behavior. *Journal of Sports Medicine and Physical Fitness, 33*(1), 83-88.

Paluch, A.E., Gabriel, K.P., Fulton, J.E., Cora E. Lewis, C.E., Schreiner, P.J., Sternfeld, B., Sidney, S.; Siddique, J., Whitaker, K.M., & Carnethon, M.R. (2021). Steps per day and all-cause mortality in middle-aged adults in the coronary artery risk development in young adults study. *JAMA Network Open, 4*(9), e2124516. https://doi.org/10.1001/jamanetworkopen.2021.24516

Rikli, R.E., & Jones, C.J. (1999). Development and validation of a functional fitness test for community-residing older adults. *Journal of Aging and Physical Activity, 7*(2), 129-161. https://doi.org/10.1123/japa.7.2.129

Vogels, E.A. (2020, January 9). About one-in-five Americans use a smart watch or fitness tracker. Pew Research Center. www.pewresearch.org/fact-tank/2020/01/09/about-one-in-five-americans-use-a-smart-watch-or-fitness-tracker

Dhingra LS, Aminorroaya A, Oikonomou EK, et al. Use of Wearable Devices in Individuals With or at Risk for Cardiovascular Disease in the US, 2019 to 2020. *JAMA Netw Open.* 2023;6(6):e2316634. doi:10.1001/jamanetworkopen.2023.16634

Brown N, Powell M, Baskin M, Oster R, Demark-Wahnefried W, Hardy C, Pisu M, Thirumalai M, Townsend S, Neal W, Rogers L, Pekmezi D

Design and Rationale for the Deep South Interactive Voice Response System–Supported Active Lifestyle Study: Protocol for a Randomized Controlled Trial

JMIR Res Protoc 2021;10(5):e29245

URL: https://www.researchprotocols.org/2021/5/e29245

DOI: 10.2196/29245

Chapter 7

Armstrong M., Paternostro-Bayles M., Conroy M.B., Franklin B.A., Richardson C., & Kriska A. (2018). Preparticipation screening prior to physical activity in community lifestyle interventions. *Transl J Am Coll Sports Med, 3,* 176–180. https://doi.org/10.1249/TJX.0000000000000073

Blair, S.N., Dunn, A.L., Marcus, B.H., Carpenter, R.A., & Jaret, P. (2001). *Active living every day.* Human Kinetics.

Canadian Society for Exercise Physiology. (2002). Physical Activity Readiness Questionnaire (PAR-Q). www.csep.ca

Doran, G.T. (1981). There's a S.M.A.R.T. way to write management's goals and objectives. *Management Review, 70*(11), 35-36.

Franklin, B.A., Thompson, P.D., Al-Zaiti, S.S., Albert, C.M. Hivert, M.-F., Levine, B.D., Felipe Lobelo, Madan, K., Sharrief, A.Z., & Eijsvogels, T.M.H. (2020). Exercise-related acute cardiovascular events and potential deleterious adaptations following long-term exercise training: placing the risks into perspective—an update: A scientific statement from the American Heart Association. *Circulation, 141,* e705-e736. https://doi.org/10.1161/CIR.0000000000000749

Chapter 8

Bandura, A. (1986). *Social foundations of thought and action: A social cognitive theory.* Prentice Hall.

Bandura, A. (1997). *Self-efficacy: The exercise of control.* W.H. Freeman.

Blair, S.N., Dunn, A.L., Marcus, B.H., Carpenter, R.A., & Jaret, P.E. (2021). *Active living every day* (3rd ed.). Human Kinetics.

Dunn, A.L., Garcia, M.E., Marcus, B.H., Kampert, J.B., Kohl, H.W., & Blair, S.N. (1998). Six-month physical activity and fitness changes in Project Active, a randomized trial. *Medicine and Science in Sports and Exercise, 30*(7), 1076-1083.

Dunn, A.L., Marcus, B.H., Kampert, J.B., Garcia, M.E., Kohl, H.W., III, & Blair, S.N. (1997). Reduction in cardiovascular disease risk factors: 6-month results from Project Active. *Preventive Medicine, 26*(6), 883-892.

Joseph, R.P., Keller, C., Adams, M.A., & Ainsworth, B.E. (2015). Print versus a culturally-relevant Facebook and text message delivered intervention to promote physical activity in African American women: A randomized pilot trial. *BMC Women's Health, 15,* 30. https://doi.org/10.1186/s12905-015-0186-1

Morrison, L., McDonough, M.H., Zimmer, C., Din, C., Hewson, J., Toohey, A., Crocker, P.R.E., & Bennett, E.V. (2023). Instructor social support in the group physical activity context: Older participants' perspectives. *Journal of Aging and Physical Activity, 31*(5), 765-775. https://doi.org/10.1123/japa.2022-0140

Pekmezi, D., Fontaine, K., Rogers, L.Q., Pisu, M., Martin, M.Y., Schoenberger-Godwin, Y.-M., Oster, R.A., Kenzik, K., Ivankova, N.V., & Demark-Wahnefried, W. (2022). Adapting MultiPLe behavior Interventions that eFfectively Improve (AMPLIFI) cancer survivor health: Program project protocols for remote lifestyle intervention and assessment in 3 inter-related randomized controlled trials among survivors of obesity-related cancers. *BMC Cancer, 22*, 471. https://doi.org/10.1186/s12885-022-09519-y

Prochaska, J.O., & DiClemente, C.C. (1983). The stages and processes of self-change in smoking: Towards an integrative model of change. *Journal of Consulting and Clinical Psychology, 51*(3), 390-395.

Rinne, M., & Toropainen, E. (1998). How to lead a group: Practical principles and experiences of conducting a promotional group in health-related physical activity. *Patient Education and Counseling, 33*(1S), S69-S76.

Pappas, S. (2023, March 1). Group therapy is as effective as individual therapy, and more efficient. Here's how to do it successfully. *Monitor on Psychology, 54*(2). https://www.apa.org/monitor/2023/03/continuing-education-group-therapy

Gentry MT, Lapid MI, Clark MM, Rummans TA. Evidence for telehealth group-based treatment: A systematic review. *Journal of Telemedicine and Telecare.* 2019;25(6):327-342. doi:10.1177/1357633X18775855

Chapter 9

Abdin, S., Welch, R.K., Byron-Daniel, J., & Meyrick, J. (2018). The effectiveness of physical activity interventions in improving well-being across office-based workplace settings: A systematic review. *Public Health, 160*, 70-76.

Brown, N.I., Powell, M.A., Baskin, M., Oster, R., Demark-Wahnefried, W., Hardy, C., Pisu, M., Thirumalai, M., Townsend, S., Neal, W.N., Rogers, L.Q., Pekmezi, D. (2021). Design and rationale for the Deep South interactive voice response system–supported active lifestyle study: Protocol for a randomized controlled trial. *JMIR Research Protocols, 10*(5), e29245. https://doi.org/10.2196/29245

Buckingham, S.A., Williams, A.J., Morrissey, K., Price, L., & Harrison, J. (2019). Mobile health interventions to promote physical activity and reduce sedentary behaviour in the workplace: A systematic review. *Digital Health, 5*. https://doi.org/10.1177/2055207619839883

Burn, N.L., Weston, M., Maguire, N., Atkinson, G., & Weston, K.L. (2019). Effects of workplace-based physical activity interventions on cardiorespiratory fitness: A systematic review and meta-analysis of controlled trials. *Sports Medicine, 49*(8), 1255-1274. https://doi.org/10.1007/s40279-019-01125-6

Clemes, S.A., O'Connell, S.E., & Edwardson, C.L. (2014). Office workers' objectively measured sedentary behavior and physical activity during and outside working hours. *Journal of Occupational and Environmental Medicine, 56*(3), 298-303. https://doi.org/10.1097/JOM.0000000000000101

Coulson, J.C., McKenna, J., & Field, M. (2008). Exercising at work and self-reported work performance. *International Journal of Workplace Health Management, 1*(3), 176-197. https://doi.org/10.1108/17538350810926534.

Dishman, R.K., Oldenburg, B., O'Neal, H., & Shephard, R.J. (1998). Worksite physical activity interventions. *American Journal of Preventive Medicine, 15*(4), 344-361.

Heise TL, Frense J, Christianson L, & Seuring, T. (2021). Using financial incentives to increase physical activity among employees as a strategy of workplace health promotion: Protocol for a systematic review. *BMJ Open, 11*, e042888. https://doi.org/10.1136/bmjopen-2020-042888

Hoenemeyer, T.W., Cole, W.W., Oster, R.A., Pekmezi, D.W., Pye, A., & Demark-Wahnefried, W. (2022). Test/retest reliability and validity of remote vs. in-person anthropometric and physical performance assessments in cancer survivors and supportive partners. *Cancers, 14*(4), 1075. https://doi.org/10.3390/cancers14041075

Jirathananuwat, A., & Pongpirul, K. (2017). Promoting physical activity in the workplace: A systematic meta-review. *Journal of Occupational Health, 59*(5), 385-393. https://doi.org/10.1539/joh.16-0245-RA

Kazi, A., Duncan, M., Clemes, S., & Haslam, C. (2014). A survey of sitting time among UK employees. *Occupational Medicine, 64*(7), 497-502.

Kohll, A. (2019, January 9). Why we pay our employees to exercise at work. *Forbes*. www.forbes.com/sites/alankohll/2019/01/09/why-we-pay-our-employees-to-exercise-at-work

MacEwen, B.T., MacDonald, D.J., & Burr, J. F. (2015). A systematic review of standing and treadmill desks in the workplace. *Preventive Medicine, 70*, 50-58.

Marcus, B.H., Emmons, K.M., Simkin-Silverman, L.R., Linnan, L.A., Taylor, E.R., Bock, B.C., et al. (1998). Evaluation of stage-matched versus standard self-help physical activity interventions at the workplace. *American Journal of Health Promotion, 12*(4), 246-253.

Marshall, A.L., Owen, N., & Bauman, A.E. (2004). Mediated approaches for influencing physical activity: Update of the evidence on mass media, print, telephone and website delivery of interventions. *Journal of Science in Medicine and Sport, 7*(Suppl.), 74-80.

Miller, R, & Brown, W. (2004). Steps and sitting in a working population. *International Journal of Behavioral Medicine, 11*(4), 219-224.

Muir, S.D., Silva, S.S.M., Woldegiorgis, M.A., Rider, H., Meyer, D., & Jayawardana, M.W. (2019). Predictors of success of workplace physical activity interventions: A systematic review. *Journal of Physical Activity & Health, 16*(8), 647-656. https://doi.org/10.1123/jpah.2018-0077

Osibanjo, R. (2022, June 30). The post-pandemic office: How to win employees back. *Forbes*. www.forbes.com/sites/richardosibanjo/2022/06/30/the-post-pandemic-office-how-to-win-employees-back

Royer, H., Stehr, M., & Sydnor, J. (2015). Incentives, commitments, and habit formation in exercise: Evidence from a field experiment with workers at a Fortune-500 company. *American Economic Journal: Applied Economics, 7*(3), 51-84.

Sharratt, M.T., & Cox, M. (1988). Employee fitness: State of the art. *Canadian Journal of Public Health, 79*(2), S40-S43.

Shephard, R.J. (1992). A critical analysis of work-site fitness programs and their postulated economic benefits. *Medicine and Science in Sports and Exercise, 24*(3), 354-370.

Shrestha, N., Kukkonen-Harjula, K.T., Verbeek, J.H., Ijaz, S., Hermans, V., & Pedisic, Z. (2018). Workplace interventions for reducing sitting at work. *Cochrane Database of Systematic Reviews, 6*(6), CD010912. https://doi.org/10.1002/14651858.CD010912.pub4

U.S. Census Bureau. (2022, September 15). The number of people primarily working from home tripled between 2019 and 2021. www.census.gov/newsroom/press-releases/2022/people-working-from-home.html

Jeroen C. M. Barte & G. C. Wanda Wendel-Vos (2017) A Systematic Review of Financial Incentives for Physical Activity: The Effects on Physical Activity and Related Outcomes, Behavioral Medicine, 43:2, 79-90, DOI: 10.1080/08964289.2015.1074880

Chapter 10

Abrams, D.B. (1991). Conceptual models to integrate individual and public health interventions: The example of the workplace. In M. Henderson (Ed.), *Proceedings of the International Conference on Promoting Dietary Change in Communities* (pp. 170-190). Fred Hutchinson Cancer Research Center.

Almeida, D.P., Alberto, K.C., & Mendes, L.L. (2021). Neighborhood environment walkability scale: A scoping review. *Journal of Transport & Health, 23*, 101261.

Atske, S., & Perrin, A. (2021, July 16). Home broadband adoption, computer ownership vary by race, ethnicity in the U.S. Pew Research Center. www.pewresearch.org/short-reads/2021/07/16/home-broadband-adoption-computer-ownership-vary-by-race-ethnicity-in-the-u-s

Auxier, B., & Anderson, M. (2021, April 7). Social Media Use in 2021: A majority of Americans say they use YouTube and Facebook, while use of Instagram, Snapchat and TikTok is especially common among adults under 30. Pew Research Center. www.pewresearch.org/internet/2021/04/07/social-media-use-in-2021

Brown, N.I., Powell, M.A., Baskin, M., Oster, R., Demark-Wahnefried, W., Hardy, C., Pisu, M., Thirumalai, M., Townsend, S., Neal, W.N., Rogers, L.Q., & Pekmezi, D. (2021). Design and rationale for the Deep South Interactive Voice Response System-Supported Active Lifestyle Study: Protocol for a randomized controlled trial. *JMIR Research Protocols, 10*(5), e29245. https://doi.org/10.2196/29245

Brown, N.I., Stewart, L., Rogers, L.Q., Powell, M.A., Hardy, C.M., Baskin, M.L., Oster, R.A., Pisu, M., Demark-Wahnefried, W., & Pekmezi, D. (2023). Assessing the built environment, programs, and policies that support physical activity opportunities in the rural Deep South. *Preventive Medicine Reports, 33*, 102223. https://doi.org/10.1016/j.pmedr.2023.102223

Cardinal, B.J., & Sachs, M.L. (1996). Effects of mail-mediated, stage-matched exercise behavior change strategies on female adults' leisure-time exercise behavior. *Journal of Sports Medicine and Physical Fitness, 36*(2), 100-107.

Centers for Disease Control and Prevention. (2011). Strategies to prevent obesity and other chronic diseases: The CDC guide to strategies to increase physical activity in the community. National Center for Chronic Disease Prevention and Health Promotion. https://stacks.cdc.gov/view/cdc/11994

Cerin, E., Saelens, B.E., Sallis, J.F., & Frank, L.D. (2006). Neighborhood Environment Walkability Scale: Validity and development of a short form. *Medicine and Science in Sports and Exercise, 38*(9), 1682-1691. https://doi.org/10.1249/01.mss.0000227639.83607.4d

de Vries, R.A.J., Truong, K.P., Zaga, C. et al. (2017). A word of advice: How to tailor motivational text messages based on behavior change theory to personality and gender. *Personal and Ubiquitous Computing, 21*, 675-687. https://doi.org/10.1007/s00779-017-1025-1

Dishman, R.K., & Buckworth, J. (1996). Increasing physical activity: A quantitative synthesis. *Medicine and Science in Sports and Exercise, 28*(6), 706-719.

Fulton, J.E., Buchner, D.M., Carlson, S.A., Borbely, D., Rose, K.M., O'Connor, A.E., Gunn, J.P., & Petersen, R. (2018). CDC's Active People, Healthy Nation: Creating an active America, together. *Journal of Physical Activity and Health, 15*(7), 469-473. https://doi.org/10.1123/jpah.2018-0249

Glanz, K., Rimer, B.K., & Viswanath, K. (2015). *Health behavior: Theory, research, and practice* (5th ed.). Wiley.

Golsteijn, R.H.J., Bolman, C., Volders, E., Peels, D.A., de Vries, H. & Lechner, L. (2018). Short-term efficacy of a computer-tailored physical activity intervention for prostate and colorectal cancer patients and survivors: A randomized controlled trial. *International Journal of Behavioral Nutrition and Physical Activity, 15*, 106. https://doi.org/10.1186/s12966-018-0734-9

Hartley, D., Yousefian, A., Umstattd, R., Hallam, J., Economos, C., Hyatt, R., & Hennessy, E. (2009). Rural Active Living Assessment (RALA) toolkit: Codebook and assessment tools. University of Southern Maine, Maine Rural Health Research Center.

Heath, G.W., Brownson, R.C., Kruger, J., Miles, R., Powell, K.E., Ramsey, C.T., & the Task Force on Community Preventive Services (2006). The effectiveness of urban design and land use and transport policies and practices to increase physical activity: A systematic review. *Journal of Physical Activity and Health, 3*(Suppl. 1), S55-S76t.

Huhman, M., Kelly, R.P., & Edgar, T. (2017). Social marketing as a framework for youth physical activity initiatives: A 10-year retrospective on the legacy of CDC's VERB campaign. *Current Obesity Reports, 6*, 101-107. https://doi.org/10.1007/s13679-017-0252-0

Humpel, N., Owen, N., & Leslie, E. (2002). Environmental factors associated with adults' participation in physical activity: A review. *American Journal of Preventive Medicine, 22*, 188-199.

Kahn, E.B., Ramsey, L.T., Brownson, R.C., Heath, G.W., Howze, E.H., Powell, K.E., Stone, E.J., Rajab, M.W., & Corso, P. (2002). The effectiveness of interventions to increase physical activity: A systematic review. *American Journal of Preventive Medicine, 22*, 73-107.

Kehl, M., Brew-Sam, N., Strobl, H., Tittlbach, S., & Loss, J. (2021). Evaluation of community readiness for change prior to a participatory physical activity intervention in Germany. *Health Promotion International, 36*(Suppl 2), ii40-ii52. https://doi.org/10.1093/heapro/daab161

King, A.C. (1998). How to promote physical activity in the community: Research experiences from the U.S. highlighting different community approaches. *Patient Education and Counseling, 33*, S3-S12.

King, A.C., Friedman, R., Marcus, B.H., Castro, C., Forsyth, L.H., Napolitano, M., et al. (2002). Harnessing motivational forces in the promotion of physical activity: The Community Health Advice by Telephone (CHAT) project. *Health Education Research* [Special issue], *17*(5), 627-636.

King, A.C., Friedman, R.H., Marcus, B.H., Castro, C., Napolitano, M., Ahn, D., & Baker, L. (2007). Ongoing physical activity advice by humans versus computers: The Community Health Advice by Telephone (CHAT) trial. *Health Psychology, 26*(6), 718-727.

King, A.C., Haskell, W.L., Taylor, C.B., Kraemer, H.C., & DeBusk, R.F. (1991). Group vs. home-based exercise training in healthy older men and women. *Journal of the American Medical Association, 266*, 1535-1542.

King, A.C., Taylor, C.B., Haskell, W.L., & DeBusk, R.F. (1988). Strategies for increasing early adherence to and long-term maintenance of home-based exercise training in healthy middle-aged men and women. *American Journal of Cardiology, 61*, 628-632.

Kotler, P., & Zaltman, G. (1971). Social marketing: An approach to planned social change. *Journal of Marketing, 35*, 3-12.

Kubacki, K., Ronto, R., Lahtinen, V., Pang, B., & Rundle-Thiele, S. (2017). Social marketing interventions aiming to increase physical activity among adults: A systematic review. *Health Education, 117*(1), 69-89.

Larsen, B., Marcus, B., Pekmezi, D., Hartman, S., & Gilmer, T. (2017). A web-based physical activity intervention for Spanish-speaking Latinas: A costs and cost-effectiveness analysis. *Journal of Medical Internet Research, 19*(2), e43. https://doi.org/10.2196/jmir.6257

Linke, S.E., Dunsiger, S.I., Gans, K.M., Hartman, S.J., Pekmezi, D., Larsen, B.A., Mendoza-Vasconez, A.S., & Marcus, B.H. (2019). Association between physical activity intervention website use and physical activity levels among Spanish-speaking Latinas: Randomized controlled trial. *Journal of Medical Internet Research, 21*(7), e13063. https://doi.org/10.2196/13063

Luepker, R.V., Murray, D.M., Jacobs, D.R., Jr., & Mittelmark, M.B. (1994). Community education for cardiovascular disease prevention: Risk factor changes in the Minnesota Heart Health Program. *American Journal of Public Health, 84*, 1383-1393.

Marcus, B.H., Banspach, S.W., Lefebvre, R.C., Rossi, J.S., Carleton, R.A., & Abrams, D.B. (1992). Using the stages of change model to increase the adoption of physical activity among community participants. *American Journal of Health Promotion, 6*(6), 424-429.

Marcus, B.H., Bock, B.C., Pinto, B.M., Forsyth, L.H., Roberts, M., & Traficante, R. (1998). Efficacy of individualized, motivationally tailored physical activity intervention. *Annals of Behavioral Medicine, 20*(3), 174-180.

Marcus, B.H., Dunsiger, S., Pekmezi, D., Benitez, T., Larsen, B., & Meyer, D. (2022). Physical activity outcomes from a randomized trial of a theory- and technology-enhanced intervention for Latinas: The Seamos Activas II study. *Journal of Behavioral Medicine, 45*, 1-13. https://doi.org/10.1007/s10865-021-00246-6

Marcus, B.H., Dunsiger, S.I., Pekmezi, D.W., Larsen, B.A., Bock, B.C., Gans, K.M., Marquez, B., Morrow, K.M., & Tilkemeier, P. (2013). The Seamos Saludables study: A randomized controlled physical activity trial of Latinas. *American Journal of Preventive Medicine, 45*(5), 598-605. https://doi.org/10.1016/j.amepre.2013.07.006.

Marcus, B.H., Dunsiger, S.I., Pekmezi, D., Larsen, B.A., Marquez, B., Bock, B.C., Gans, K.M., Morrow, K.M., & Tilkemeier, P. (2015). Twelve-month physical activity outcomes in Latinas in the Seamos Saludables trial. *American Journal of Preventive Medicine, 48*(2), 179-182. https://doi.org/10.1016/j.amepre.2014.08.032.

Marcus, B.H., Emmons, K.M., Simkin-Silverman, L.R., Linnan, L.A., Taylor, E.R., Bock, B.C., et al. (1998). Evaluation of stage-matched versus standard self-help physical activity interventions at the workplace. *American Journal of Health Promotion, 12*(4), 246-253.

Marcus, B.H., Hartman, S.J., Pekmezi, D., Dunsiger, S.I., Linke, S.E., Marquez, B., Gans, K.M., Bock, B.C., Larsen, B.A., & Rojas, C. (2015). Using interactive Internet technology to promote physical activity in Latinas: Rationale, design, and baseline findings of Pasos Hacia la Salud. *Contemporary Clinical Trials, 44*, 149-158. https://doi.org/10.1016/j.cct.2015.08.004.

Marcus, B.H., Lewis, B.A., Williams, D.M., Dunsiger, S I., Jakicic, J.M., Whiteley J.A., Albrecht, A.E., Napolitano, M.A., Bock, B.C., Tate, D.F., Sciamanna, CA., & Parisi, A.F. (2007). A comparison of Internet and print-based physical activity interventions. *Archives of Internal Medicine, 167*(9), 944-949.

Marcus, B.H., Napolitano, M.A., King, A.C., Lewis, B.A., Whiteley, J.A., Albrecht, A.E., Parisi, A.F., Bock, B.C., Pinto, B.M., Sciamanna, C., Jakicic, J.M., & Papandonatos, G.D. (2007). Telephone versus print delivery of an individualized motivationally tailored physical activity intervention: Project STRIDE. *Health Psychology, 26*(4), 401-409.

Marcus, B.H., Nigg, C.R., Riebe, D., & Forsyth, L.H. (2000). Interactive, preventive communication strategies: A proactive approach for reaching out to large populations. *American Journal of Health Promotion, 19*(2), 121-126.

Marcus, B.H., Owen, N., Forsyth, L.H., Cavill, N.A., & Fridinger, F. (1998). Physical activity interventions using mass media, print media, and information technology. *American Journal of Preventive Medicine, 15*(4), 362-378.

Marshall, A.L., Owen, N., & Bauman, A.E. (2004). Mediated approaches for influencing physical activity: Update of the evidence on mass media, print, telephone and website delivery of interventions. *Journal of Science, Medicine, & Sport, 7*(Suppl.), 74-80.

McLeroy, K.R., Bibeau, D., Steckler, A., & Glanz, K. (1988). An ecological perspective on health promotion programs. *Health Education Quarterly, 15*(4), 351-377.

Mendoza-Vasconez, A.S., Benitez, T., Dunsiger, S., Gans, K.M., Hartman, S.J., Linke, S.E., Larsen, B.A., Pekmezi, D., & Marcus, B.H. (2022). Pasos Hacia la Salud II: Study protocol for a randomized controlled trial of a theory- and technology-enhanced physical activity intervention for Latina women, compared to the original intervention. *Trials, 23*(1), 621. https://doi.org/10.1186/s13063-022-06575-4

Odukoya, O., Molobe, I., Olufela, O., Oluwole, E., Yesufu, V., Ogunsola, F., & Okuyemi, K. (2023). Exploring church members' perceptions towards physical activity, fruits and vegetables consumption, and church's role in health promotion: Implications for the development of church-based health interventions. *Journal of Public Health in Africa, 14*(1), 2112. https://doi.org/10.4081/jphia.2023.2112

Pekmezi, D., Ainsworth, C., Desmond, R., Pisu, M., Williams, V., Wang, K., Holly, T., Meneses, K., Marcus, B., & Demark-Wahnefried, W. (2020). Physical activity maintenance following home-based, individually tailored print interventions for African American women. *Health Promotion Practice, 21*(2), 268-276. https://doi.org/10.1177/1524839918798819

Pekmezi, D.W., Neighbors, C.J., Lee, C.S., Gans, K.M., Bock, B.C., Morrow, K.M., Marquez, B., Dunsiger, S., & Marcus, B.H. (2009). A culturally adapted physical activity intervention for Latinas: A randomized controlled trial. *American Journal of Preventive Medicine, 37*(6), 495-500. https://doi.org/10.1016/j.amepre.2009.08.023

Pellerine, L.P., O'Brien, M.W., Shields, C.A., Crowell, S.J., Strang, R., & Fowles, J.R. (2022). Health care providers' perspectives on promoting physical activity and exercise in health care. *International Journal of Environmental Research and Public Health, 19*(15), 9466. https://doi.org/10.3390/ijerph19159466

Romeo, A., Edney, S., Plotnikoff, R., Curtis, R., Ryan, J., Sanders, I., Crozier, A., & Maher, C. (2019). Can smartphone apps increase physical activity? Systematic review and meta-analysis. *Journal of Medical Internet Research, 21*(3), e12053. https://doi.org/10.2196/12053

Saelens, B.E., Sallis, J.F., Black, J.B., & Chen, D. (2003). Neighborhood-based differences in physical activity: An environment scale evaluation. *American Journal of Public Health, 93*, 1552-1558. https://doi.org/10.2105/AJPH.93.9.1552

Schmid, K.L., Rivers, S.E., Latimer, A.E., & Salovey, P. (2008). Targeting or tailoring? Maximizing resources to create effective health communications. *Marketing Health Services, 28*(1), 32-37.

Short, C.E., James, E.L., Girgis, A., D'Souza, M.I., & Plotnikoff, R.C. (2015). Main outcomes of the Move More for Life trial: A randomised controlled trial examining the effects of tailored-print and targeted-print materials for promoting physical activity among post-treatment breast cancer survivors. *Psycho-Oncology, 24*(7), 771-778. https://doi.org/10.1002/pon.3639

Stoddard, A.M., Palombo, R., Troped, P.J., Sorensen, G., & Will, J.C. (2004). Cardiovascular disease risk reduction: The Massachusetts WISEWOMAN project. *Journal of Women's Health* (Larchmont), *13*(5), 539-546.

Thirumalai, M., Brown, N., Niranjan, S., Townsend, S., Powell, M.A., Neal, W., Schleicher, E., Raparla, V., Oster, R., Demark-Wahnefried, W., & Pekmezi, D. (2022). An interactive voice response system to increase physical activity and prevent cancer in the rural Alabama Black belt: Design and usability study. *JMIR Human Factors, 9*(1), e29494. https://doi.org/10.2196/29494

U.S. Department of Health and Human Services, Public Health Service, Centers for Disease Control and Prevention, National Center for Chronic Disease Prevention and Health Promotion, & Division of Nutrition and Physical Activity. (1999). *Promoting physical activity: A guide for community action.* Human Kinetics.

Will, J.C., Farris, R.P., Sander, C.G., Stockmyer, C.K., & Finklestein, E.A. (2004). Health promotion interventions for disadvantaged women: Overview of the WISEWOMAN projects. *Journal of Women's Health* (Larchmont), *13*(5), 484-502.

Xia, Y., Deshpande, S., & Bonates, T. (2016). Effectiveness of social marketing interventions to promote physical activity among adults: A systematic review. *Journal of Physical Activity and Health, 13*(11), 1263-1274. https://doi.org/10.1123/jpah.2015-0189

Young, D.R., Haskell, W.L., Taylor, C.B., & Fortmann, S.P. (1996). Effect of community health education on physical activity knowledge, attitudes, and behavior. *American Journal of Epidemiology, 144*(3), 264-274.

Yousefian, A., Hennessy, E., Umstattd, M.R., Economos, C.D., Hallam, J.S., Hyatt, R.R., & Hartley, D. (2010). Development of the rural active living assessment tools: Measuring rural environments. *Preventive Medicine, 50*(Suppl 1), S86-S92. https://doi.org/10.1016/j.ypmed.2009.08.018

Sallis JF, Johnson MF, Calfas KJ, Caparosa S, Nichols JF. Assessing perceived physical environmental variables that may influence physical activity. *Res Q Exerc Sport.* 1997 Dec;68(4):345–351

Pekmezi DW, Neighbors CJ, Lee CS, Gans KM, Bock BC, Morrow KM, Marquez B, Dunsiger S, Marcus BH. A culturally adapted physical activity intervention for Latinas: a randomized controlled trial. Am J Prev Med. 2009 Dec;37(6):495-500. doi: 10.1016/j.amepre.2009.08.023. PMID: 19944914; PMCID: PMC2814545.

Amy V. Ries, Shira Dunsiger, Bess H. Marcus, Physical activity interventions and changes in perceived home and facility environments, Preventive Medicine,Volume 49, Issue 6, 2009, Pages 515-517, ISSN 0091-7435, https://doi.org/10.1016/j.ypmed.2009.10.009.

Goethals, L., Barth, N., Hupin, D. *et al.* Social marketing interventions to promote physical activity among 60 years and older: a systematic review of the literature. *BMC Public Health* **20**, 1312 (2020). https://doi.org/10.1186/s12889-020-09386-x

Noar SM, Benac CN, Harris MS. Does tailoring matter? Meta-analytic review of tailored print health behavior change interventions. Psychol Bull. 2007 Jul;133(4):673-93. doi: 10.1037/0033-2909.133.4.673. PMID: 17592961.

Kreuter, M., Farrell, D., Olevitch, L., & Brennan, L. (2000). *Tailoring health messages: Customizing communication with computer technology.* Lawrence Erlbaum Associates Publishers.

Kreuter, M. W., & Holt, C. L. (2001). How do people process health information? Applications in an age of individualized communication. *Current Directions in Psychological Science, 10*(6), 206–209. https://doi.org/10.1111/1467-8721.00150

Rimer BK, Orleans CT, Fleisher L, Cristinzio S, Resch N, Telepchak J, Keintz MK. Does tailoring matter? The impact of a tailored guide on ratings and short-term smoking-related outcomes for older smokers. Health Educ Res. 1994 Mar;9(1):69-84. doi: 10.1093/her/9.1.69. PMID: 10146734.

Joseph RP, Durant NH, Benitez TJ, Pekmezi DW. Internet-Based Physical Activity Interventions. Am J Lifestyle Med. 2014 Jan;8(1):42-68. doi: 10.1177/1559827613498059. PMID: 25045343; PMCID: PMC4103664.

Williams V, Brown N, Becks A, Pekmezi D, Demark-Wahnefried W. Narrative Review of Web-based Healthy Lifestyle Interventions for Cancer Survivors. Ann Rev Res. 2020;5(4):555670. doi: 10.19080/arr.2020.05.555670. Epub 2020 Mar 10. PMID: 33294850; PMCID: PMC7720895.

Pekmezi D, Ainsworth C, Joseph RP, Williams V, Desmond R, Meneses K, . . . Demark-Wahnefried W. (2017). Pilot Trial of a Home-based Physical Activity Program for African American Women. *Med Sci Sports Exerc, 49*(12), 2528–2536. doi: 10.1249/MSS.0000000000001370

INDEX

Note: The italicized *f* and *t* following page numbers refer to figures and tables, respectively.

A

abstinence violation effect 35
accelerometers 77-80, 78*f*, 81
Active Living Every Day 61, 129
activity trackers. *See* time tracking methods; specific types
aerobic physical activity 4
analyzer role 118, 119*t*
appraising 48
assessment. *See* physical activity assessment; physical fitness assessment; readiness assessment

B

backsliding, in physical activity habits 14
barriers to physical activity
    in decision-making theory 30-31, 31*f*, 49-50
    group stage-specific strategies for 133-134
    IDEA approach to 96-98, 97*f*
    individual stage-specific strategies for 103, 104-105, 107, 109, 111
    lack of time 73
    in marketing community programs 158
    psychological readiness 92-96, 93*f*, 95*f*, 96*f*
    social disparities 7
behavioral choice theory 31-33, 32*f*, 36*t*
behavioral processes of change
    described 17, 17*t*-18*t*
    measuring 43-45, 44*t*-45*t*
    in sample group curriculum 125*t*, 126-129, 127*t*
behavior change, influences on 11, 12*f*. *See also* mediators of change; processes of change
Behavior Change Wheel 36-37
behavior goals 123-124. *See also* goal setting and planning
benefits of physical activity
    in decision-making theory 30-31, 31*f*, 49-50
    in individual stage-specific strategies 103, 104, 106, 109, 111
    list of 3-4
    marketing community programs and 158
    in psychological readiness assessment 95, 95*f*
    selling worksite programs and 140
books and articles (resource list) 189-190
Borg Rating of Perceived Exertion 73
bouts of activity 4-5, 6

C

caffeine, and heart rate 83, 84
cardiovascular disease risk 90, 153
CBPR (community-based participatory research) 25-26, 36*t*
change. *See* mediators of change; processes of change; theoretical models
cognitive process of change
    described 17, 17*t*-18*t*
    measuring 43-45, 44*t*-45*t*
    in sample group curriculum 125*t*, 126-129, 127*t*
communication channels
    in community programs 162-165, 166-174
    print versus telephone 62-63
    text messages 63-64, 64*t*
    in worksite programs 139, 142, 148-149, 150
community-based participatory research (CBPR) 25-26, 36*t*
community norms 11, 12*f*, 157
community programs
    case example 159
    community leaders role in 165
    Jump Start to Health study 59-60
    Project Active 61-62, 125*t*, 126
    Project Stride 62-63
    readiness assessment 154-157, 155*f*
    remote delivery of 162-165
    Seamos Activas studies 61, 63-64
    stage-specific strategies for 165-174
    Step Into Motion study 64-65
    target audience 153-154, 158
    targeted and tailored approaches to 160-162, 160*f*, 161*f*
confidence (self-efficacy)
    defined 45
    individual stage-specific strategies for 105, 107, 109, 112
    measuring 46-47, 98-99
    in social cognitive theory 27, 45-46
confidence (self-efficacy) questionnaire 46-47, 181
Conquering Mount Everest event 149
consultant role 118, 119*t*
counseling. *See* group counseling; intervention programs; individual counseling
curriculum sample, for groups 125*t*, 126-129, 127*t*
cyclical nature of stages 13-14, 13*f*

D

daily physical activity, defined 5-6. *See also* physical activity
decisional balance 30, 31*f*, 49-50
decisional balance questionnaire 50, 183-184

211

decision-making theory 30-31, 31*f*, 36*t*
DiClemente, C. 11
diffusion of innovations (DOI) 26
doing some physical activity (stage 3) 13, 15*t*. *See also* stages of motivational readiness for change model; stage-specific strategies

E

ecological model 23-24, 24*t*, 36*t*
emotional support 48
emotions, and heart rate 84
employees. *See* worksite programs
enjoyment of physical activity 51-53
enjoyment of physical activity scale 52-53, 186
environmental factors in physical activity
    community environments 25*t*, 154, 155*f*, 156-157
    worksite environments 138-139
etapas de cambio (stages of change) questionnaire 177
events, event planning
    community programs 167, 169, 171, 172, 174
    worksite programs 144-145, 147, 148, 149
exercise, defined 5. *See also* physical activity

F

Facebook groups 126
facilitator role 118, 119*t*
feedback to clients 59-60
fitness trackers 77-80, 78*f*, 139
flowchart for determining stage of change 19*f*
four P's of marketing 158

G

goal setting and planning
    in community programs 157
    in group counseling 123-125
    in individual counseling 100-101, 100*f*, 101*f*
    individual stage-specific strategies for 103, 105, 107-108, 109-110, 112-113
    role in behavior change 47
    step counting goals 76, 77*f*
group counseling
    benefits and types of 117-118
    case example 128
    goal setting in 123-125
    group size and duration 121
    leader effectiveness 129-130
    leader's roles and teaching styles 118, 118*t*-119*t*
    no-show clients 121-122
    sample curriculum 125*t*, 126-129, 127*t*
    session format for 124-125
    social support in 120-121
    stage-specific strategies for 130-135
    virtual 117, 122-123, 126
group leaders
    effectiveness assessment 129-130
    roles and teaching styles 118, 118*t*-119*t*
group participation
    group stage-specific strategies for 131-133
    worksite incentives 145

H

health risk screening 89-92, 91*f*
heart rate monitoring
    resting heart rate 83-84, 84*f*
    target heart rate 72-73
history of physical activity questionnaire 92, 187
home-based workers 138
hybrid workers 138

I

IDEA problem-solving technique 96-98, 97*f*
individual counseling
    case example 113-114
    gauging client confidence 98-99
    goal setting in 100-101, 100*f*, 101*f*
    IDEA technique in 96-98, 97*f*
    measuring successes 102
    physical readiness assessment 89-92, 91*f*
    psychological readiness assessment 92-96, 93*f*, 95*f*, 96*f*
    stage-specific strategies for 102-113
    virtual 115
individual influence on behavior 11, 12*f*
individual-level theories
    versus interpersonal 26
    origins and guiding principles 28-35
    social cognitive theory 26-28
informational social support 48
information dissemination
    community stage-specific strategies for 166, 168, 170, 171-172, 173
    group stage-specific strategies for 132-133, 134-135, 168
    in worksite 139
institutional factors in physical activity 11, 12*f*, 154, 155*f*
instrumental support 48
intensity of physical activity
    determining level of 71-73
    examples by activity 71*t*
    levels and recommendations 4-5
    in worksite programs 144
Internet-based intervention 64-65, 164-165
interpersonal influence on behavior 11, 12*f*
interpersonal-level theories
    versus individual 26
    origins and guiding principles 28-35
intervention programs. *See also* community programs; group counseling; worksite programs; individual counseling
    communication channels in 62-64, 64*t*
    design of 7-8
    individual feedback in 59-60
    Internet-based 64-65

lifestyle approach to 61-62
muscle-strengthening in 62
stage-matched 15-16, 18
stage-matched materials for 58-59, 142-143
technology-enhanced 63-64, 64*t*
theory-based 41-43, 41*f*
for underserved populations 60-61

J
Jump Start to Health study 58-60

L
lapse versus relapse 35
leaders of stage-based groups
　effectiveness assessment 129-130
　roles and teaching styles 118, 118*t*-119*t*
learning theory 28-30, 28*f*, 36*t*
legislation and policies 11, 12*f*, 157
levels of influences on behavior 11, 12*f*, 24*t*. *See also* mediators of change; processes of change
lifestyle approach to exercise 61-62
light activity 79
long-term goals 100, 100*f*

M
making physical activity a habit (stage 5) 13, 15*t*. *See also* stages of motivational readiness for change model; stage-specific strategies
management support of worksite programs 139-140
manuals and materials, stage-matched 58-59, 142-143
marketing, in community programs 158, 159
mass media 166, 168
mediators of change. *See also* processes of change
　considering in program design 39-43
　decisional balance 30, 49-50
　defined 39, 55
　enjoyment of physical activity 51-53
　goal setting and planning 47
　versus moderators 53-54
　outcome expectations 27, 51
　self-efficacy 27, 45-47
　social support 48-49
meeting physical activity guidelines (stage 4) 13, 15*t*. *See also* stages of motivational readiness for change model; stage-specific strategies
metabolic disease 90
mobile apps 74, 79, 139
moderate-intensity activities
　defined 4
　examples of 5, 71*t*
　as worksite program focus 144
moderators, versus mediators 53-54
motivational readiness for change model. *See* stages of motivational readiness for change model

motivator role 118, 118*t*-119*t*
muscle-strengthening activities 5, 62

N
neighborhood environments 25*t*, 154, 155*f*
Neighborhood Environment Walkability Scale 156
no-show clients, in groups 121-122
not thinking about change (stage 1) 12, 15*t*. *See also* stages of motivational readiness for change model; stage-specific strategies

O
office workers, as sedentary 137
organizations (resource list) 189
outcome expectations 27, 51
outcome expectations for exercise scale 51, 185

P
PAR-Q (Physical Activity Readiness Questionnaire) 91-92, 91*f*
Pasos Hacia la Salud study 42-43, 65
patterns of physical activity behavior 70
pedal exercisers, under-desk 139
pedometers 30, 75, 81
pen and paper activity tracking 80, 80*f*
perceived exertion 73
physical activity. *See also* barriers to physical activity; benefits of physical activity
　benefits list 3-4
　defined 5-6
　enjoyment of 51-53
　influences on 24*t*, 25*t*, 154, 155*f*
　recommendations for 4-5, 6
physical activity assessment
　behavior patterns 70
　exercise intensity 71-73
　time tracking 73-82, 76*f*, 77*f*, 80*f*
physical activity awareness
　community stage-specific strategies for 165-167
　worksite stage-specific strategies for 146-147
physical activity enjoyment scale 52-53, 186
physical activity history questionnaire 92, 187
physical activity interventions. *See* intervention programs
physical activity maintenance
　community stage-specific strategies for 173-174
　group stage-specific strategies for 134-135
　individual stage-specific strategies for 111-113
　worksite stage-specific strategies for 150, 151-152
Physical Activity Readiness Questionnaire (PAR-Q) 91-92, 91*f*
physical activity stages of change questionnaire
　form 176
　use of 20, 70, 140
physical fitness, defined 5

physical fitness assessment
   importance of 83
   resting heart rate 83-84, 84f
   two-minute step test 86-87
   walking test 84, 85f
physical readiness assessment. *See* readiness assessment
planning. *See* goal setting and planning
PPA (Program and Policy Assessment) 156-157
print material, in interventions 62-63, 162-163
problem-solving technique 96-98, 97f
processes of change
   measuring 17, 43-45, 44t-45t
   in sample group curriculum 125t, 126-129, 127t
   stages of change and 16
   types of 17, 17t-18t
processes of change questionnaire 17, 178-180
process goals 123-124. *See also* goal setting and planning
Prochaska, J. 11
Program and Policy Assessment (PPA) 156-157
Project Active 61-62, 125t, 126
Project Stride 62-63
prompts and reminders 30
psychological readiness
   assessment of 94-96, 95f, 96f
   as barrier to activity 92
   IDEA approach to 96-98, 97f
   individual stage-specific strategies for 103-113
   past successful changes and 93-94, 93f
public policy 11, 12f, 157
pulse, finding on wrist 83

Q

questionnaires 175-187
   confidence (self-efficacy) 181
   decisional balance 50, 183-184
   etapas de cambio (stages of change) 177
   outcome expectations scale 51, 185
   PAR-Q 91-92, 91f
   physical activity enjoyment scale 52-53, 186
   physical activity history 92, 187
   processes of change 178-180
   social support scale 49, 182
   stages of change 20, 70, 140, 176

R

rating of perceived exertion 73
readiness assessment
   for community programs 154-157
   individual stage-specific strategies for 102-113
   initial physical screening 89-92, 91f
   physical activity history 92
   psychological readiness 92-98, 93f, 95f, 96f
   for worksite programs 140-141

readiness to change model. *See* stages of motivational readiness for change model
reciprocal determinism 26, 27f
recruitment, in worksite programs 141-142
relapse prevention model 33-35, 34f, 36t
reminders and prompts 30, 79, 139
remote interventions
   community 162-165
   group 117, 122-123, 126
   individual 115
remote workers 138
renal disease 90
resource list 189-190
resting heart rate 83-84, 84f
rewards, in learning theory 29
Rogers, Everett 26

S

Seamos Activas studies 61, 63-64
sedentary lifestyle 3, 7, 57, 137
self-efficacy. *See* confidence (self-efficacy)
self-regulation skills 47
shaping 28-29
short-term goals 100, 100f
sitting alerts 30, 79
SMART goals 101, 101f, 124. *See also* goal setting and planning
smart phone apps 74, 79, 139
smart watches 78f, 79
smoking, and heart rate 83, 84
social cognitive theory 26-28, 36t, 46
social disparities 7
social marketing 158, 159
social media groups 126
social networks, in community assessment 157
social support
   in group counseling 120-121
   measuring 49
   types and sources of 48-49
social support for physical activity scale 49, 182
societal factors in physical activity 154, 155f
SSA (Street Segment Assessment) 156-157
stage-based group curriculum 125t, 126-129, 127t
stage-matched materials and messages
   community programs 160-162, 160f, 161f
   worksite programs 58-59, 142-143
stages of change questionnaire. *See also* etapas de cambio (changes of stage) questionnaire
   form 176
   use of 20, 70, 140
stages of motivational readiness for change model
   cyclical nature of 13-14, 13f
   determining client's readiness stage 18-20, 19f
   development of 11
   stages in 12-13, 15t
   treatment strategies and 15-16, 18

stage-specific strategies. *See also* intervention programs
   community programs 165-174
   group counseling 130-135
   individual counseling 102-113
   worksite programs 145-152
standing desks 139
step counting
   devices for 75
   goals for 76, 77*f*
   step counter log 76*f*
Step Into Motion study 64-65
stimulants, and heart rate 83, 84
Street Segment Assessment (SSA) 156-157
strength training 5, 62
stress management, in workplace 140
success, meauring
   individual stage-specific strategies for 103-104, 106, 108, 110, 113
   methods of 102
suggested reading 189-190

T

tailored approach 160-162, 160*f*, 161*f*
Take a Walk in My Shoes event 148
talk test 72
target audience
   community programs 153-154, 158
   worksite programs 141-142
targeted approach 160-162, 160*f*, 161*f*
target heart rate 72-73
telephone, in interventions 62-63, 163-164
termination stage 14
text messages, in interventions 63-64, 64*t*
theoretical models. *See also* stages of motivational readiness for change model
   behavioral choice theory 31-33, 32*f*
   community-based participatory research 25-26
   decision-making theory 30-31, 31*f*
   diffusion of innovations 26
   ecological model 23-24, 24*t*
   as intervention basis 41-43, 41*f*
   learning theory 28-30, 28*f*
   overview of 36*t*
   readiness for change 8-9
   relapse prevention model 33-35, 34*f*
   social cognitive theory 26-28
thinking about change (stage 2) 12, 15*t*. *See also* stages of motivational readiness for change model; stage-specific strategies
time, as physical activity barrier 73
time tracking methods
   accelerometers 77-80, 78*f*
   pedometers 75
   pen and paper 80, 80*f*
   recommending to clients 81-82
   step counter log 76*f*
   step goal chart 77*f*
   weekly report example 82*f*
Top 10 Benefits T-Shirt Contest 147
Town-Wide Assessment (TWA) 156-157
transtheoretical model. *See* stages of motivational readiness for change model
treadmill desks 139
treatment strategies and programs. *See* intervention programs
T-Shirt Contest, Top 10 Benefits 147
TWA (Town-Wide Assessment) 156-157
two-minute step test 86-87

U

under-desk pedal exercisers 139
underserved populations 60-61
unmotivated clients 40

V

vigorous-intensity activities 4, 5, 71*f*
virtual interventions
   community 162-165
   group 117, 122-123, 126
   individual 115

W

walking
   in community goals 157
   for meeting physical activity guidelines 6
   as moderate-intensity activity 4, 144
   during workday 139
walking test 84, 85*f*
wearable devices
   accelerometers 77-80, 81
   fitness tracker use 78*f*
   pedometers 75, 81
   as reminders 30
web sites (resource list) 190
working from home 138
worksite programs
   activity intensity and liability 144
   activity-oriented environments 138-139
   communication channels in 139, 142, 148-149, 150
   event planning 144-145
   Jump Start to Health study 58-59
   need for 137
   participation incentives 145
   readiness assessment 140-141
   for remote workers 138
   selling to management 139-140
   stage-matched materials for 142-143
   stage-specific strategies for 145-152
   target audience recruitment 141-142

ABOUT THE AUTHORS

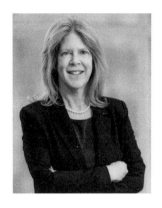

Bess H. Marcus, PhD, is a professor of behavioral and social sciences and dean emerita of the School of Public Health at Brown University. She was professor and chair of the department of family medicine and public health at the University of California San Diego from 2011-2017. She is a clinical health psychologist who has spent over 30 years conducting research on physical activity behavior and has published over 300 papers and book chapters as well as three books on this topic. She has developed a series of assessment instruments to measure psychosocial mediators of physical activity behavior and has also developed low-cost interventions to promote physical activity behavior in community, workplace, and primary care settings. Dr. Marcus is actively involved on numerous NIH grants on physical activity behavior and public health. Her work increasingly focuses on promoting physical activity in underserved and vulnerable populations. She has mentored numerous students, post-doctoral fellows, and faculty. She is the recipient of numerous awards including the Citation Award from the American College of Sports Medicine (ACSM) in 2015. She delivered the President's Lecture at the 2015 ACSM meeting and the Morris/Paffenbarger Exercise is Medicine Lecture at the 2022 meeting.

Marcus enjoys staying active by daily walks with family and friends. She also enjoys strength training, yoga, and Pilates.

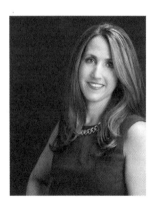

Dori Pekmezi, Ph.D., is a licensed clinical psychologist and professor and vice chair in the department of health behavior in the School of Public Health at the University of Alabama at Birmingham. Her research and teaching focus on the application of behavioral theory and technology to physical activity promotion in underserved or at-risk populations. She has published over 100 professional articles and book chapters on these topics and served as principal investigator or co-investigator on at least 15 physical activity research grants. Pekmezi is also a fellow of the Society of Behavioral Medicine and served as cochair for the professional society's Physical Activity Special Interest Group.

Dr. Pekmezi stays physically active by playing tennis with her friends and walking her sons to school.